Health Technology Assessments and Rare Diseases

PHARMACEUTICALS POLICY AND LAW

Pharmaceuticals Policy and Law

Volume 13

Earlier published in this series

Vol.1. J.L. Valverde and G. Fracchia (Eds), Focus on Pharmaceutical Research
Vol.2. J.L. Valverde (Ed), The Problem of Herbal Medicines Legal Status
Vol.3. J.L. Valverde (Ed), The European Regulation on Orphan Medicinal Products
Vol.4. J.L. Valverde (Ed), Information Society in Pharmaceuticals
Vol.5. C. Huttin (Ed), Challenges for Pharmaceutical Policies in the 21st Century
Vol.6. J.L. Valverde and P. Weissenberg (Eds), The Challenges of the New EU Pharmaceutical Legislation
Vol.7. J.L. Valverde (Ed), Blood, Plasma and Plasma Proteins: A Unique Contribution to Modern Healthcare
Vol.8. J.L. Valverde (Ed), Responsibilities in the Efficient Use of Medicinal Products
Vol.9(1,2). J.L. Valverde (Ed), 2050: A Changing Europe. Demographic *Crisis* and Baby Friend Policies
Vol.9(3,4). J.L. Valverde (Ed), Key Issues in Pharmaceuticals Law
Vol.10. J.L. Valverde and D. Watters (Eds), Focus on Immunodeficiencies
Vol.11(1,2). J.L. Valverde and A. Ceci (Eds), The EU Paediatric Regulation
Vol.11(3). J.L. Valverde (Ed), Health Fraud and Other Trends in the EU
Vol.11(4). J.L. Valverde (Ed), Rare Diseases: Focus on Plasma Related Disorders
Vol.12(1,2). J.L. Valverde and A. Ceci (Eds), Innovative Medicine: The Science and the Regulatory Framework
Vol.12(3,4). J.L. Valverde (Ed), New Developments of Pharmaceutical Law in the EU
Vol.13(1,2). J.L. Valverde (Ed), Challenges for the Pharmaceuticals Policy in the EU

Health Technology Assessments and Rare Diseases

Pharmaceuticals Policy and Law
Volume 13, 2011

Editors

J.L. Valverde
Chair Jean Monnet, Granada, Spain
and
J. Prevot
International Patient Organisation for Primary Immunodeficiencies, Cornwall, UK

IOS Press

Amsterdam • Washington, DC • Tokyo

ISBN 978-1-60750-982-0

Publisher
IOS Press
Nieuwe Hemweg 6B
1013 BG Amsterdam
The Netherlands
fax: +31 20 687 0019
e-mail: order@iospress.nl

Distributor in the UK and Ireland
Gazelle Books
Services Ltd.
White Cross Mills
Hightown
Lancaster LA1 4XS
United Kingdom
fax: +44 1524 63232
e-mail: sales@gazellebooks.co.uk

Distributor in the USA and Canada
IOS Press, Inc.
4502 Rachael Manor Drive
Fairfax, VA 22032
USA
fax: +1 703 323 3668
e-mail: iosbooks@iospress.com

Printed in the Netherlands

PHARMACEUTICALS POLICY AND LAW
Volume 13(3,4), 2011

CONTENTS

5. Industry perspectives

6. HTA perspectives

7. Glossary

Appendices

Pharmaceuticals Policy and Law 13 (2011) 115–116
DOI 10.3233/PPL-2011-0317
IOS Press

Editorial

Health Technology Assessments (HTAs) in Europe and similar assessment procedures in other regions such as comparative effectiveness in the United States, are increasingly being used to measure the clinical efficacy and cost effectiveness of health technologies. Ultimately these mechanisms are also in place to control healthcare budget expenditure.

The topic of HTAs has become in recent years increasingly debated in various international fora and it has become obvious that in order for such processes to be transparent, unbiased and carried out in a robust manner, the involvement of key stakeholders such as patient organization representatives, physicians, health economists and industry representatives amongst others is absolutely necessary.

This is particularly relevant in the case of rare diseases therapies. There are indeed many hurdles that come into play when assessing rare diseases therapies such as the unavailability of Randomised Clinical Trials (RCTs) due to the small patient populations and the seemingly high cost of such therapies.

This edition of *Pharmaceuticals Policy and Law* seeks to provide an international overview of these challenges by outlining the viewpoints of key expert stakeholders in the field.

It is hoped that these perspectives will enrich and contribute to the current discussions both at the level of EU institutions and in the United States as well as to the initiatives of platforms such as HTAi and EUnetHTA and other involved organizations. Particularly the need to involve stakeholders and look beyond medical and cost effectiveness factors to include the societal impact of health technologies in the HTA process.

We also hope that the book will be valuable to any person wishing to better understand the issues surrounding the use of HTAs and similar mechanisms in the assessment of rare diseases therapies and will contribute to a better awareness of the key factors that need be taken into account into such processes.

We are grateful to the numerous participating authors including HTA specialist theorists, health economists, patient organizations, rare diseases umbrella organizations, stakeholder platforms, physicians, HTA agency representatives and industry who accepted to present their perspectives on this important topic.

Pharmaceuticals Policy and Law wishes to thank vividly all authors that have made this monograph possible. With our special thanks to the European Commissioner for Health, Mr. John Dalli, for endorsing this important topic and for highlighting the key European health policy developments and initiatives in the Foreword to this volume.

Jose-Luis Valverde
Editor-in-Chief
Pharmaceuticals Policy and Law

Johan Prevot
Co-Editor
Executive Director,
International Patient
Organisation for Primary
Immunodeficiencies (IPOPI)

Pharmaceuticals Policy and Law 13 (2011) 117–120
DOI 10.3233/PPL-2011-0318
IOS Press

Foreword

John Dalli
European Commissioner for Health and Consumer Policy, Brussels, Belgium

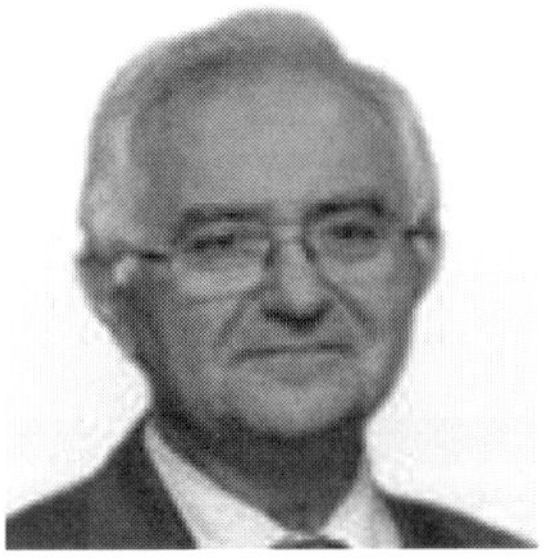

I welcome this new series on *"Health Technology Assessments and Rare Diseases Therapies"*. As the use of health technology assessment increases, this is an important opportunity to reflect on the progress that can be made at European level to help the many millions of sufferers of rare diseases in Europe.

Currently, between 5 000 and 8 000 different rare diseases affect around 6–8% of the total EU population, or around 29–36 million Europeans. The relatively limited number of patients affected by specific rare diseases, and the fragmentation of knowledge about them, makes this a prime example where working at European level is not only beneficial, but even necessary.

The European Commission is playing an active role by helping patients to receive appropriate and timely diagnosis, information and care by supporting Member States in their efforts to work together and pool their knowledge, expertise and resources in this important area.

Support for EU-wide cooperation on health technology assessment has been ongoing for over five years. For example, EU funding has helped to establish a European network linking HTA agencies. Within this network, a common methodological approach to HTA has been developed. This model simplifies the re-use of HTA information made in one country and offers the potential for task-sharing between Member States. This is clearly more efficient than each Member State working in isolation.

European Reference Networks

We hope to build on this valuable work with the newly adopted **EU Directive on the application of patients' rights in cross-border healthcare (Directive 2011/24/EU).**

The Directive foresees the development of **European Reference Networks** and the adoption of criteria and conditions that healthcare providers should fulfil in order to be part of those networks.

Such networks should have the capacity to provide complex or highly technological diagnostic or treatment services for medical conditions requiring a particular concentration of expertise, resources or technology, as is the case for many rare diseases.

This would improve access to high quality and highly specialised expertise across Europe enabling the mobility of medical expertise, particularly when patient or professional mobility is not possible.

EU cooperation on HTA

Currently, the EU co-finances formal intergovernmental co-operation on HTA involving almost all Member States. Through this cooperation, HTA agencies will use the "HTA core model" they have developed to assess different kinds of health technologies. By testing this model through a significant number of pilots, we will gain important insights into how Member States can cooperate most effectively in this field.

From 2013 onwards, HTA co-operation will move from *a project-driven* to a *regular* network. The EU Directive on patients' rights in cross-border healthcare defines HTA as one of the key areas for co-operation between Member States. The European Commission's ambition is that the future HTA network should establish both costeffective and time-effective ways to cooperate on HTA. This could result in less duplication of work between Member States when assessing the clinical effectiveness of health technologies. It could also benefit companies as it establishes more common standards for industry submissions for reimbursements in Member States. And most importantly, it could benefit the patients by providing broad and timely access to valuable health technologies.

National Plans and strategies on rare diseases

In parallel, Member States are elaborating – and some have already adopted – national plans or strategies on rare diseases. The European Commission-funded EUROPLAN Project (European Project for Rare Diseases National Plans Development) provides valuable support to Member States to set out clear guidelines, indicators and content for their national plans. The project will be further developed through formal intergovernmental cooperation which is expected to be launched later this year, with the clear objective of providing technical assistance and training for Member States.

Investment for the future

The visibility and inventorying of rare diseases still need to be improved. This is why the European Commission launched another Joint Action last year to support and broaden the ORPHANET database, the world reference database on rare diseases. The European Commission has so far funded this database with €6 million so that rare diseases are adequately coded and traceable in all health information systems. Any patient or health professional can receive information on all the clinics, hospitals and specialists able to treat the disease in all EU Member States. It also provides information on orphan medicines currently available, ongoing clinical trials, best practices, information on patients' organisations and registers. Information on 5 868 rare diseases are already available on this database.

The European Union is also a major funder of research on rare diseases. The main financing instrument for research at EU level is the 7th Research Framework Programme covering the period 2007–2013. It has so far invested €75 million in 20 research projects on rare diseases across the EU.

Empowerment

To succeed in any policy on rare diseases we need to listen and learn from patients themselves. Member States are encouraged to closely consult patients' representatives on policy development; facilitate patients' access to updated information on rare diseases; and promote the important activities of patients' organisations. For its part, the European Commission has been working closely for many years with organisations such as EURORDIS, the European organisation representing patients of rare diseases, and will continue to do so.

Solutions

The area of rare diseases is clearly one where assessing new treatments is particularly challenging. The low number of patients at Member State level makes it difficult for manufacturers of new medicines to make optimal clinical studies. HTA agencies similarly straggle to assess new treatments where few or no alternatives exist. As a consequence, it often takes time before Member States make decisions on the use and reimbursement of new rare disease treatments.

Rare diseases is therefore an area where increased EU cooperation is essential. Cooperation may increase the total number of patients available to participate in research and development of new treatments. This equally applies to HTA as joint approaches to assessing treatments for rare disease patients can allow for better access to patients' data.

To explore these possibilities, rare disease medicines could be among those piloted in further formal inter-governmental cooperation on HTA.

Earlier this year, the European Commission commissioned a study by Ernst & Young to explore mechanisms for a more effective introduction of orphan medicines onto the markets of EU Member States. This study will look at the different actors involved in the process leading to an orphan medicine being given to a patient – such as the European Medicines Agency, HTA agencies and national health insurers.

It will suggest alternative and/or improved mechanisms for better co-ordination between all actors involved in the process. Ibis is particularly pertinent considering that today, it often takes too much time at national level to decide on the actual use or non-use of a new orphan medicine following the marketing authorisation given by the European Commission. The study will be finalised later this year. On the basis of this study, the Commission will consider if further action is required.

EU initiatives on rare diseases can support increased EU-wide cooperation on HTA and improved treatment and hence a better quality of life for rare disease patients all over Europe.

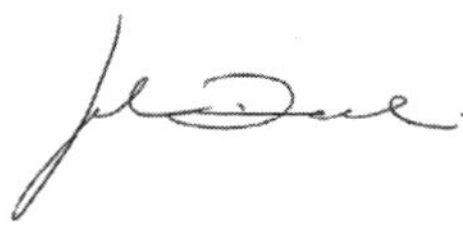

1. Introduction

Pharmaceuticals Policy and Law 13 (2011) 123–128
DOI 10.3233/PPL-2011-0319
IOS Press

Patient aspects and involvement in HTA: An academic perspective

Helle Ploug Hansen[a,*] and Anne Lee[b]
[a] *Institute of Public Health, Man and Society & National Research Centre for Cancer Rehabilitation, University of Southern Denmark, Odense, Denmark*
[b] *Centre for Applied Health Services Research and Technology Assessment, University of Southern Denmark, Odense, Denmark*

There is an increasing focus on designing health services that are 'patient focussed'. This is also reflected in health technology assessment (HTA), with a growing emphasize on patient perspectives and involvement. The purpose of this article is to discuss why and how patient aspects may be addressed in future HTAs'. While involving patients in the HTA process we argue that the assessments of the included aspects must be based in research to provide both relevant and valid results that can inform health policy decision makers. Patient aspects need to be explored when a technology, the organisation and/or economic aspects of a technology affect and influence patients in one way or another. "Patients" are in this sense understood as; any current or potential health service user or beneficiary of a health technology, and since illness and the use of technology often involves the family, their perspectives may also be included.

When exploring patient aspects in relation to the use of technology it is necessary to reflect on the modes of knowledge. It is important that researchers bear in mind that their understanding of knowledge always have implications in relation to the validity and scope of the research results, they produce.

Keywords: Patient aspects, qualitative methodology, object-knowledge, relational-knowledge

1. Introduction

There is an increasing focus on designing health services that are "patient focussed", including involvement of patients in decision-making about health care services and delivery. This general focus is also reflected in health technology assessment (HTA), with growing emphasize on the assessment of patient aspects in relation to the technology being assessed, as well as towards patient's involvement in the HTA process [1]. While the involvement of patients in the HTA process is still somehow incipient, there is in Denmark a long tradition for including patient aspects in the assessments. HTAs are most often conducted within a framework of four key elements: technology, patient, organization, and economy. In the recently updated Danish Handbook of HTA [2], it is stated that the patient element must focus on the assessment of *patient aspects*, such as patient perspectives, needs, experiences,

*Corresponding author: Helle Ploug Hansen, Institute of Public Health, Research Unit: Health, Man and Society & National Research Centre for Cancer Rehabilitation, University of Southern Denmark, J.B. Winsløwsvej 9b, Odense, Denmark. Tel.: +45 65502989; E-mail: hphansen@health.sdu.dk.

preferences and acceptance of a given technology. In relation to these aspects the handbook emphasizes theoretical considerations concerning modes of knowledge and the production of knowledge. Furthermore, it pays a close attention to the use of qualitative methodology in order to assess patient aspects, for example using in-depth interviews, focus groups and/or participant-observation.

A review on the inclusion of patient and/or organizational aspects in HTA reports published by INATHA members 2000–2005 showed that just 38% of the reports included one or both of the two aspects. Less than half of the reports, including patient aspects, stated research questions specific for the patient aspects. The review showed a great variation in relation to how profound the issues included were assessed, and in how explicit methodological considerations were reported e.g. why and how the issues were included and addressed [3,4]. In a forthcoming article, a review of the Danish tradition of including a specific patient focussed element is presented [5]. The review shows that patient aspects were included in 58 of 62 Danish HTA reports published between 1999 and 2010. Of the 58 reports; 93% included objectives and/or research questions for the assessments of patient aspects, and 59% included patient aspects in the final recommendations of the report [5]. This indicates that Danish HTA reports, to a greater extent than most, include patient aspects and does it in a considered manner. We argue that this finding demonstrates that inclusion of patient aspects in HTAs' to a high degree depends on institutional awareness and interest in these issues.

In this article we define the term "patient"; as broad term meaning any current or potential health service user or beneficiary of a health technology [1]. The purpose is to discuss why and how patient aspects can be addressed in future HTAs'. Our approach is academic. We argue that assessments of patient aspects must be based in research and scientific approaches to provide robust and valid results that can inform health policy decision makers [1]. While experienced in HTA, we have not researched rare diseases within HTAs'. However, we argue that the scientific approach of investigating patient aspects within the context of rare diseases is similar to that of other diseases.

2. Why and when to include patient aspects in an HTA?

No doubt the aim of including patient aspects and involve them in an HTA must be to develop new knowledge, and to make sure that the knowledge produced is both scientifically robust and relevant for the specific group of patients. Our point of departure is that the patients are the ones experiencing the full path of disease and treatment. Patients' have personal, bodily, social and cultural experiences, understandings and practices in relation to coping with illnesses and the use of technology. At the same time they act as patients, consumers, members of families, communities, and as citizens in the society. Furthermore, the illnesses and the use of technology do not only affect the patient but very often also the significant other(s) being; husbands, wife's, children, parents, friends, informal caregivers etc. This may especially be the case for people experiencing rare diseases which often are genetic, lifelong and may occur in early childhood [6]. Patients and their significant others can therefore provide important information, exceeding clinical and economic effectiveness such as views and experiences about how daily life is affected by illness and the use of health technologies. A few examples are; an article on fathers coping with their newborn being screened and diagnosed with cystic fibrosis [7] an article on young adults' perceptions of living with cystic fibrosis and its treatment during the transition to adulthood [8] and an article on how individuals with genetic conditions learn about, live with and manage their conditions [9].

We claim that patient aspects need to be explored and patients need to be involved when a technology, the organisation and/or economical aspects of a technology affect and influence patients in one way or another. And since a (health) technology seldom does anything by it itself, this means nearly allways.

Our perception of health technology is in line with the Science and Technology Studies described by Pascale Lehoux [10] among others. In that understanding a technology does not work or produce effect in isolation from the people (patients, health care professionals, researchers, politicians, decision-makers) handling the technology. It is in a clinical, social, cultural, organizational and economic context that a specific technology is shaped and re-shaped. This happens by the ways in which the people actual use and interpret the technology [[10], chapter 2]. In other words, a technology does not by itself improve for example a patient's health status or quality of life. It is also in the hands of the patients to act with a technology (to take a tablet, participate in a screening programme, perform training exercise after operation, etc.) Thereby a patient can be seen as a co-producer of a given technology and of the kind of change that the utilization of the technology might produce.

3. How to grasp and how to understand?

Research and research findings entails a specific understanding of knowledge and knowledge production which can either be empirically, theoretically or politically based. Understandings of knowledge can be explicitly expressed or implicitly embedded in a study. An analysis of the patient element in a Danish HTA-report concerning "Patient education" demonstrates for example; that the decision of using secondary research in form of a systematic literature review, instead of using primary research (through either surveys, interviews, focus groups, participant-observation etc.) was not discussed, and the move from the HTA questions to the search criteria, particular search categories, words and their combination were not set out explicitly [11]. However, search procedures, inclusions and exclusions have implications for the literature found and for what counts as knowledge.

Attention to two modes of knowledge can help us to determine what kind of knowledge we need to produce in a specific HTA. Kirsten Hastrup a Danish anthropologist distinguishes between what she calls; *object*-knowledge and *relational*-knowledge [12]. In her reflections on knowledge and evidence in anthropology she makes several important points relevant for our purpose. Hastrup states that; "Knowledge must be organized information. The organization implies that knowledge is both reductive and selective. It is reductive because it renders empirical complexity and messiness in clear, but therefore also more limited propositions about the world. It is selective, because for it to be knowledge it has to disregard some information" [12, p. 456].

3.1. Object-knowledge

This mode of knowledge, also described as "encyclopedic knowledge" [12] consists in largely ontological propositions about for example health, diseases, health systems, nature etc. The most common methods used to gain object-knowledge are clinical examinations (e.g. blood tests, x-rays etc.) and quantifying data from registers and surveys. One example from the field of rare diseases therapy is a study of cognitive rehabilitation in relation to people with Multiple Sclerosis. In this study the technology, a highly standardized rehabilitation program, was validated through changes in brain activity measured by Functional Magnetic Resonance Imagining. In the study a specific pattern of brain activity was seen as a measurement for cognition [13]. The example demonstrates how the knowledge produced becomes *an object* – something that we can observe, possess, accumulate and recycle. Object-knowledge is "fact" oriented and detached from the influence of social relations, time and space and may therefore be seen, as Lehoux puts it "generally falling short of providing an in-depth understanding of what technologies do in practice" [9, p. 41]. We argue that object-knowledge is important but also has considerable limitations. It cannot stand alone when wanting to explore and understand patient aspects, or when wanting to involve patients in an HTA.

3.2. Relational-knowledge

"This mode of knowledge consists in propositions about knowledge as *relational*. It attaches itself to relations between people or between people and objects and it emerges within a dialogical field" [12, p. 456]. This understanding of knowledge implies that "knowing is a matter of perspective; There is no knowledge without someone *who knows* in a particular way. Knowledge therefore is a social phenomenon rather than simply a substance" [12, p. 456]. The knowledge that patients' produce and reproduce about the day-to-day reality of living with the condition (a rare disease for example) is not so much "fact and object" knowledge as it is "relational" knowledge. It becomes produced in the dialogical fields of living in families, being a child going to school, being an adult going to work, coping with illness and its treatments. One example from the field of rare diseases therapy is a study of the role of gender and coping in relation to parents of children with high functioning autism or Asperger's syndrome [14]. In this study a qualitative analysis based on in-depth interviews demonstrated the various strategies that parents use to cope with their child's disability and how these strategies were constructed and reconstructed in the context of the family, economy and the wider social context [14].

The most common methods used to gain relational knowledge are qualitative such as interviews, focus groups and fieldwork with participant-observations. Because of the often small number of patients with a specific rare disease, the use of technological facilities e.g. internet and chat rooms as well as the research methods of "synthesising qualitative studies" seem to be valuable methods.

4. How about the future?

It is of extremely importance that researchers bear in mind that their understanding of knowledge always have implications in relation to the validity and scope of the research results, they produce. Involving patients, generating HTA questions, as well as the employment of theories and methodologies to answer them, are either explicitly or implicitly informed by theoretical and methodological movements in the field of health policy research and HTA. Furthermore, it also becomes a result of the composition of the project group with respect to academic background. If health policy and decision making in relation to rare diseases is to be *patient-focused*, it is important to fully acknowledge the integrating of patient aspects in all parts of the HTA; economy, technology, organizational, ethichal and not least in the recommendations. For this to happen there must be a an awareness of the value of doing so, as well as scientifically solid evidence, available or generated through primary and/or secondary research, and in relation to the specific technology. This means that researchers in different fields will have to work more closely together doing interdisciplinary research producing both object-knowledge and relational-knowledge.

Involving patients and patient aspects in the HTA process might strengthen the production of both object- knowledge and relational-knowledge, and influence what technologies are considered relevant for an HTA as well as; what kind of problems to address, or for which to develop new technologies, or new ways of using existing technologies.

References

[1] K. Facey et al., Patients' perspectives in Health Technology Assessments: A route to robust evidence and fair liberation, *Int J Technol Assess Health Care* **26** (2010), 334–340.

[2] F.B. Kristensen and H. Sigmund, eds, *Health Technology Assessment Handbook*, Danish Centre for Health Technology Assessment, National Board of Health, 2007.

[3] National Board of Health, Danish Centre for Health Technology Assessment, *A Review of Organisational and Patient-Related Assessments in HTAs Published by INAHTA*, members, Copenhagen: National Board of Health. Danish Centre for Health Technology Assessment, 2007.

[4] A. Lee, L.S. Skött and H.P. Hansen, Organizational and patient-related assessments in HTAs: state of the art, *Int J Technol Assess Health Care* **25**(4) (2009), 530–536.

[5] H.P. Hansen, A. Lee and C.B.V. Randwijk, Patient aspects. A review of 58 Danish HTA reports, *Int J Technol Assess Health Care* (2011).

[6] K. Facey, Patient involvement in HTA: what added value? *Pharmaceuticals Policy and Law* **13** (2011), 245–251,

[7] L. Priddis, J. Dunwoodie, E. Balding, A. Barrett and T. Douglas, Paternal experiences of their children's diagnosis of Cystic Fibrosis following newborn screening diagnosis, *Neonatal, Paediatric & Child Health Nursing* **13**(2) (Jul 2010), 4–10.

[8] J.M. Berge, J.M. Patterson, D. Goetz and C. Milla, Gender differences in young adults' perceptions of living with cystic fibrosis during the transition to adulthood: a qualitative investigation, *Families, Systems & Health: The Journal of Collaborative Family HealthCare* **25**(2) (Jun 2007), 190–203.

[9] A. Petersen, The Best Experts: The Narratives of Those Who Have a Genetic Condition, *Social Science & Medicine* **63**(1) (2006), 32–42.

[10] P. Lehoux, *The Problem of Health Technology*, Policy implications for modern Health Care Systems. Routledge 2006

[11] T. Tjørnhøj-Thomsen and H.P. Hansen, How, who and what: an investigation of patient aspects in health technology assessments, *Int J Technol Assess Health Care* (2011).

[12] K. Hastrup, Getting it right: Knowledge and evidence in anthropology. Sage Publications, London 2004. (http://ant.sagepub.com/).

[13] J. Sastre-Garriga, J. Alonso, M. Renom, M.J. Arévalo, I. González, I. Galán, X. Montalban and A. Rovira, A functional magnetic resonance proof of concept pilot trial of cognitive rehabilitation in multiple sclerosis, *Mult Scler* **17** (2011), 457. Originally published online 21 December 2010. DOI: 10.1177/1352458510389219.

[14] D.E. Gray, Gender and Coping: the parents of children with high functioning autism, *Soc Sci & Med* **56** (2003), 631–642.

Pharmaceuticals Policy and Law 13 (2011) 129–160
DOI 10.3233/PPL-2011-0320
IOS Press

An introduction to key concepts in health economics for haemophilia organisations

Brian O'Mahony
Chief Executive, Irish Haemophilia Society, Dublin, Ireland

1. Introduction

The Global economic difficulties of the past five years have resulted in an increased focus on health economics, cost effectiveness analysis, cost benefit analysis and indicators examining the use of resources in health care. Health Technology Assessments (HTA) are the most widely used tool in Europe to measure the cost effectiveness of medical treatment. In the United States, Comparative Effectiveness Research (CER) is most often used. These trends are unlikely to change. I am sure that there will be increased scrutiny on the cost of healthcare, specific interventions and routine treatment for rare diseases into the future. Rare diseases are often more expensive to treat than conditions with a higher incidence. There will almost inevitably be more work done by HTA agencies and other Government bodies in examining the costs of care for rare disorders in the future. Patient organisations who represent those with rare diseases need to embrace this reality, engage positively with the process, understand the scientific data, collaborate in the production of treatment and outcome data and ensure that their voices are formally heard as an integral part of the process. The information in this chapter specifically relates to HTA's in haemophilia. However, the approach taken, the focus on the data required in any given situation and the response required is an approach which can be taken by any patient organisation dealing with any condition and more specifically with any rare disease.

People with haemophilia require lifelong treatment with clotting factor in order to manage frequent bleeding episodes and reduce the risk of joint damage requiring surgery and/or resulting in restricted mobility (as well as other potential organ damage). The prevention of bleeds with factor concentrate has become standard practice for the treatment of haemophilia. To date there have been few restrictions on funding and access to new treatments for haemophilia in developed countries. However, a climate change is occurring in haemophilia as new expensive products come to market, health care payers turns to questions of whether costs can be controlled without major detriment to patients. As a result, the areas of Health Technology Assessment (HTA) and evidence based medicine are increasing efforts to collect data on patient health outcomes and quality of life in haemophilia, and starting to assess the cost-effectiveness of treatments with the aim to control costs into the future. This trend will be exacerbated with the future introduction of longer acting factor concentrates which may have an entirely different cost base and calculation.

It is challenging to apply health economics to haemophilia due to the relative rarity of the disease (although it is more common than many other rare diseases), limits to data available (although this is changing as the need for outcomes evidence increases), and the fact that it affects children and family as well as adults. Haemophilia patient organisations need to develop at least a basic understanding of the economics of haemophilia care and the methodology and terminology associated with this. HTAs in Haemophilia will only occur in some countries but in every country haemophilia patient organisations need to prepare to deal with economic data and arguments.

The aim of this chapter is to

- Develop an understanding of the economics of Haemophilia treatment
- Develop an understanding of the Health Technology Assessment (HTA) process and its terminology
- Increase the skills of haemophilia organisations in advocating on issues relating to the economics of haemophilia care
- Identify areas where haemophilia organisations can make contributions to the HTA process
- Identify the challenges in applying the HTA process to haemophilia.

This chapter may also be useful for patients and patient organisations living in countries where HTA processes are not well developed. With the current very difficult economic situation globally projected to continue into the future, national haemophilia patient organisations and clinicians need to develop a greater appreciation of the economics of haemophilia care. The open ended provision of sufficient replacement therapy which has become the norm in many countries may be more difficult to sustain in the absence of proactive collection of evidence based data by clinicians and experiential data by patient organisations. In our separate or joint advocacy and lobbying activities in the coming years, economics will be an increasingly important criteria. We need to understand these concepts, have the ability to collect, collate and interpret the relevant data and understand the economic concepts we will be challenged with in working to improve or maintain therapy. The sort of experience-based information that patients and patient organisations contribute to HTA processes can also be useful in raising public awareness about the impact of treatment for haemophilia and the need for effective prevention and treatment. It can help make the case for better treatment in a variety of settings such as media campaigns and lobbying, or in individual consultations with doctors.

Most EU and European countries now have HTA agencies (Listed in Appendix 1). HTAs will increasingly be used not only to evaluate new technologies or therapies but to make decisions on allocation of scarce resources for the treatment of many conditions using existing therapies. Health authorities to date have generally carried out HTAs where the therapy is used by many people in a country (such as Statins to lower Cholesterol or therapies for diabetes) and therefore has a place in the list of most expensive drugs. Haemophilia is a relatively rare disorder and the cost of treatment for those with severe haemophilia is relatively high, therefore Haemophilia is now starting to appear on the radar screen of HTA agencies. In Sweden, for example, a HTA on Haemophilia is currently underway. This is not entirely surprising as Factor VIII concentrate is the third most expensive therapeutic product in Sweden -first being a therapy for Rheumatoid Arthritis and second test strips for diabetes (personal communication- Swedish Haemophilia Society) If we look specifically at Sweden as an example, HTAs have been completed in the following areas: Migraine, Diseases caused by excess stomach acid, Asthma, COPD and coughs, Hypertension, Depression and Lipid disorders. There are ongoing reviews on therapies for Diabetes, Rheumatism, Incontinence and prostate disorder, Painkillers and anti-inflammatory medications

Given the relatively high cost of therapy and the fact that several of the very widely used drugs and therapies used by the population have already been the subject of HTA's, it is not a major surprise that the HTA authority in Sweden is now examining Haemophilia. As part of the process the Swedish Haemophilia clinicians have compiled a compendium of evidence based data in haemophilia [1] which will have utility in many countries and ads to the body of evidence for optimum care. In Belgium in the list of the twenty five most expensive therapies, FVIII was classified at number eight.

In this chapter, several of the concepts discussed are illustrated using the example of Prophylaxis in haemophilia. This example has not been chosen at random. Prophylaxis for children with severe Haemophilia is recognised as the optimum standard of care by, among others, the European Association for Haemophilia and allied disorders [2], the Medical and Scientific Council of the National Hemophilia Foundation in the USA, the United Kingdom Haemophilia Doctors Organisation and the Canadian Association of Haemophilia treaters. A widely quoted randomised clinical trial in 2007 – the Joint Outcome Study [3] also supports this therapy. However, the therapy is relatively expensive when compared to on-demand therapy and therefore it is beginning to be examined with regard to cost effectiveness by health funding agencies. In particular, the continuation of prophylactic therapy into adulthood will be scrutinised. It is an area of acknowledged clinical benefit yet financial vulnerability. For these reasons we will use it as an example.

2. HTA and advocacy

Does this mean that decisions on provision of care should be taken away from clinicians and exclude also a meaningful role for patients and patient organizations?

Should we now conclude that health economists should decide which treatments are provided based solely on measured economic criteria?

The answer to both questions is a resounding No. There are many layers in decision making and different rationales for therapy. A HTA or economic assessment is but one o f these.

The rationale for effective treatment for Haemophilia are multiple:

- Haemophilia is a rare genetic condition where therapy is available which can transform the quality of life and indeed the very survival of the individual. In the absence of good therapy, the child is facing inevitable bleeding, joint damage, and perhaps early death. The adult, if he has survived faces arthropathy, pain, loss of mobility and inability to contribute fully to society.
- Adequate therapy allows the individual to treat bleeding early or ideally avoid bleeding by use of prophylactic therapy. This helps to prevent joint damage in most individuals, avoid arthropathy and allows the individual to gain an education, work, and raise and support a family. The individual can contribute fully to society. There are many genetic or serious conditions where such a positive outcome is not even remotely possible, irrespective of any therapies which may be available
- Provision of unsafe therapy in the past led to the infection of thousands of people with haemophilia with HIV, Hepatitis B and Hepatitis C. Thousands have died. This catastrophe has resulted in an enormous human cost. It has also resulted in a very high financial cost for treatment, hospitalization, compensation and inquiries. We should not allow health economists or Governments to forget the high cost of providing unsafe or sub standard treatment.
- Any individual can be born with a rare or expensive to treat condition. Considerations of equity and fairness should dictate in a reasonable society that individuals and families are not punished because of this. A survey among taxpayers in Sweden [4], for example, clearly demonstrated that when Haemophilia and the benefits of therapy were explained to them, they were willing to pay a multiple of the actual cost for both prophylaxis and on-demand therapy required for those with haemophilia. This solidarity should be an important aspect of society.
- Health economists obviously make judgements solely on economic grounds based on whether the benefits of a therapy or procedure are considered to justify the costs (with benefits typically measured in QALYs in many countries). Processes such as HTAs examine the evidence based data to support therapy and demand a high degree of evidence which they can use to predict utility values and QALYs to allow them to make judgements on cost effectiveness of therapies. However, it should be remembered that the methodologies they use to measure utility values are themselves very subjective. Techniques described later including Time Trade off, Standard gamble or Visual Analogue scale are based generally on the subjective opinion of those who are asked the questions. Generic utility questionnaires are even more subjective given the fact that the rating tables are based on the subjective opinions of people not affected by the

condition. For example, if a person with haemophilia completes an EQ5D questionnaire, the utility value this gives you is based on a time trade off exercise which has been conducted among members of the public with limited or no specific knowledge about haemophilia.. This scale is devised from asking a group of individual's questions about conditions they themselves do not suffer from.

- HTA assessments provide a guide for health authorities on the relative cost effectiveness of a medical intervention or treatment. The authorities may accept this and base their decision on this. However, this is not necessarily the case. The authorities may take a different view. In Sweden, the HTA assessment on therapy for Phenylketonuria was favourable and the cost was lower than the generally accepted Swedish cut off cost for a therapy. Despite this, the HTA finding was not implemented and the therapy has not been approved. In Ireland, a HTA on the provision of HPV vaccination for girls to prevent cervical cancer showed a relatively low cost per QALY but this was not approved and the vaccination programme was not initiated. This decision has now been re-visited following successful advocacy.
- If Haemophilia care is subjected to a HTA in a country, an unfavourable decision is not necessarily going to be implemented. The normal methods of advocacy and lobbying of Government would continue to apply. However, it would obviously be better if the HTA outcome was favourable. The possibility of a favourable outcome is enhanced if the clinicians and the national haemophilia patient organization understand the process and participate from the earliest possible stage in the process.

3. Health Technology Assessment

Health Technology Assessment is a term used to cover any aspect of healthcare from prevention programmes to devices to drugs and procedures. The aim of a Health Technology Assessment (HTA) is to examine the short and long-term consequences of using a healthcare technology. It takes into consideration the medical, social, economic and ethical issues related to the use of a health technology. The process aims to apply a systematic, transparent and unbiased approach when dealing with health technologies. HTA is used differently across Europe. In some countries, such as England and Wales, it is used to guide decisions about whether treatments and other technologies should be available on the National Health Service, based on a judgement of whether they provide value for money. In other countries the focus may be less on value for money and more on evidence of effectiveness and cost effectiveness.

A HTA can provide information to support decisions about priorities in healthcare or specific decisions about whether new treatments should be introduced, for example:

- Health authorities thinking of putting in place screening programmes;

- Health care payers deciding which technologies (e.g., operations, drugs) should be paid for;
- Health care organisations deciding whether to exclude or implement new treatments
- Health care companies producing new products (e.g. to demonstrate a level of benefit for the product that justifies the cost. A future relevant example may be long acting factor concentrates).

4. Key concepts in health economics and cost-effectiveness

Health economics is concerned with the utilisation of the insufficient resources in society to pay for all treatments and interventions that improve health such as money, time of health professionals, etc. For example, the amount of money is limited by a budget, but the amount of a nurse's time is limited by the working hours in a day. More nurses could be employed but the demand for healthcare will always outweigh the supply of such resources. Therefore, this leads to a selection process by which some treatments and patient groups receive resources and others do not, notionally termed as rationing of healthcare resource use. Rationing (or resource allocation) can be determined by using criteria such as age or ability to pay, or first come first served principle. Health economics and cost-effectiveness analysis aid rationing decisions primarily according to 'efficiency' criteria. The principle of efficiency is not about minimising costs but about allocating the resources available for treatments to produce the maximum benefit. This is not used to discriminate between individuals but to maximize overall welfare in a society. To achieve this aim health economists use cost-effectiveness analysis to identify which treatments produce the greatest population benefits for the resources available.

Cost-effectiveness analysis is used to determine 'value': the value of the resources (both paid and unpaid) used to provide treatment and care, and the value of the health benefits to a population of patients generated by this treatment. The nurse or doctors time used to treat a haemophilia patient can be simply valued according to the market salary paid for that time. However, the time spent by a child with haemophilia and the family member transporting the patient for treatment is not paid, but has a value (for example, value of time lost from school or work). A treatment, such as home treatment, that can reduce these costs by allowing the doctor or nurse to perform other tasks and/or reducing patient/family absenteeism from school/work has a value that can offset additional costs associated with the price of the treatment. Likewise, the benefits in health related quality of life associated with the control of a bleeding episode has a value to the person with haemophilia and to others including family members. It is the purpose of cost-effectiveness analysis to quantify the value of these costs and benefits. The key issue and controversy over this concerns what should be included within the value framework for the economic evaluation. This is considered further later in this chapter.

Whilst health economics is primarily about value and efficiency one further key concept to introduce is equity (justness and fairness). A treatment deemed not cost-effective may still be selected if society places an extra value on the benefits because of who (or how many) experience the health improvement. For example, people in a society may consider it fair that children or those at the end of life have a greater access to treatments and associated health benefits than other segments of the population. Also in many countries an additional value is placed on the benefits from orphan or ultra-orphan drugs for rare conditions. Patient organisations working in haemophilia have a lot of experience regarding ensuring just and fair access to effective treatments and hence can contribute to ensuring equity factors are considered within any assessment of the cost-effectiveness of haemophilia treatments.

5. Patient and patient organisation contribution to health technology assessment

It should be noted that even if the HTA process has a negative result then this evidence can be used to appeal the findings by making a case to the government. A HTA is not a decision, it only informs the decision making process

5.1. Why patient experience is important

Although HTA's are used as a method of controlling costs spent on healthcare, the results of the HTA generally do not affect the politician or decision maker. The real affects are felt by the patients, caregivers and in a wider sense the public in general. Therefore, it is essential that the patient perspective is considered in the HTA process.

HTA agencies collect all the available scientific data they believe needed to make the decision and as a result the reality of the illness on a day to day basis can be missed. The only way for the real impact of living with a condition to be understood is for the patients and patient organisations themselves to provide evidence. For example:

- Describing treatment regimes in terms of annual number of bleeds with on demand therapy versus prophylaxis may be part of the evidence based data examined. However it is meaningless unless they know what a bleed actually is. Explain what this means in reality. Describe the degree of pain experienced with an untreated bleed into a joint. Describe the inevitable long term effects of repeated bleeds into joints or muscles. Point out the very real possibility of life or limb threatening bleeds. Point out the real consequences for everyday life such as -you cannot manage to go to work/school, or you have to get your wife/partner to help you get dressed. Generally the quality of life utility value using an EQ-5D survey is assessed as being between 0 and 1 with 0 being death and 1 being perfect health. However, some health states can result in a negative

value. In Ireland, the author carried out an EQ –5D survey with 3 persons with Haemophilia. The first individual was treated with factor concentrate regularly to prevent bleeding episodes. His utility value was 1. The second individual had, at the time of the survey, a bleeding episode in his knee. His utility value was 0.587. The third individual had a serious and painful bleed in his ileo psoas muscle, His utility value was –0.095. This illustrates the impact of a single bleeding episode which may not be readily apparent in larger studies
- Record the amount of time that was missed from work/school over a year. Note if you are planning to take time out for an operation due to joint damage etc and time for hospital appointments. Also note the time you have had problems at the weekend and had to rest and miss activities with the family.
- Describing the effect a treatment has on your daily life – such as, 'it allows my child to sleep over at a friend's house and not be afraid".

It is the effect of the illness and treatment on all aspects of life that is one of the reasons that evidence from patients and the public is so important. It is important to remember that the patient and the patient organisation should focus their efforts on their needs rather than advocating for a specific product or treatment.

5.2. Patient evidence

Different HTA agencies have different ways in which they will accept patient evidence. Most have a panel that a patient and the patient organisation will meet with and discuss the important aspects of patient needs. There are two main ways in which patient evidence can be used to contribute to a HTA. The first is through the patient and caregivers talking individually about their own lives and how the illness affects them on day to day basis. This can humanise the condition for the HTA panel. It is important to choose individuals who are able to make their message understood by academic and other professional experts. Deliver the two or three key messages you want to deliver at the beginning and then elaborate with illustration of the points and return to reinforce them at the end of your allotted time. This type of presentation should be factual, anecdotal with real case examples and non emotional. An example would be the quality of life of one individual in Germany who recorded an 86% decrease in bleeding episodes in the year following his switch to a prophylactic treatment regime [5].

Patient evidence might include:

- The impact of a bleed -Short or long term
- A description of symptoms
- Symptoms that are difficult to live with

The limitations it imposes on:

- Daily life
- Ability to work

- Social life
- Enjoyment of family and friends
- The impact on a person's mental wellbeing
- Activities which people living with the illness find difficult
- Whether the illness prevents people from fulfilling their chosen role in life
- Degree of pain due to the bleeding episodes and joint damage
  * How the pain interferes with daily activities
  * Whether pain medication needs to be taken regularly
- The aspect of the illness that patients find most difficult

The second way in which patient evidence can be accepted by the HTA agency is through the patient organisation/ haemophilia society. The patient organisation should start developing evidence through qualitative research, which describes views and opinions. Patient organisations may also gather statistical data or quantitative research. The patient organisation can group trends and an overall picture that an individual cannot present. Considering the cost of haemophilia treatment this information is not only valuable in preparation for a HTA it is also extremely useful when advocating to governments on any aspect of Haemophilia care in which economic considerations may play a role..

Patient organisations should survey members, carers, doctors and these surveys might include areas such as:

For a HTA on a proposed new therapy:

- What patients and carers expect from a new treatment
- What benefits the treatment brings
- How the benefits compare with those of existing treatments

For a HTA on existing therapy:

- How it helps affected people fulfil their chosen role in life
- How important the benefits are to the patient
- The outcomes from treatment they value the most
- How the benefits impact on patients' daily life
- What unwanted effects the treatment causes such as risk of inhibitors
  * How the unwanted effects compare with those of other treatments
  * How the unwanted effects are balanced against the potential benefit
- What would happen to patients if there was limited or no access to the treatment
- How patients and carers value the treatment
- How easily the treatment fits into patients' daily life
- What is the impact on a person's psychosocial wellbeing?
- The financial impact of the technology
  * Cost of travel to hospital

    * Loss of earnings
    * Cost of paying a carer
    * Financial impact on the individual and family (for example if a child is denied access to optimal treatment, a parent may have to give up work to look after the child)

- The carer's needs

    * Taking time off work to care for the person
    * Paying for a carer for the patient
    * Paying for childcare because the patient cannot look after the child/children
    * Financial hardship because they reduce their working hours
    * Watching the patient/child suffer

6. Patient involvement

Patient involvement should be evident in all stages of the HTA process. However the mechanism for this involvement will differ between HTA agencies. Some HTA agencies will proactively seek the views of the relevant national patient organisation early in the process. Others will not seek this but will be open to representation being made by patient organisations. It is important that you ascertain the mechanism for involvement with the HTA agency in your country prior to a HTA commencing on an aspect of Haemophilia care. Do not wait until it is too late. Find out from your HTA agency which are their priority areas for examination in the coming year or years. If they are intending to examine any aspect of haemophilia care, get involved early. Contact the agency and ensure they know that you wish to make a submission. Put this request in writing. If they refuse to hear your submission, the evidence that you had requested the opportunity to make a submission and had been refused will be a strong advocacy tool in any subsequent campaign against a negative result. Ideally, get involved at an early enough stage to allow your organisation to positively influence the specific areas to be examined. If you can influence the questions, you will increase the probability that you will have an influence on the outcome. The sooner there is patient involvement in the process, the better. Getting involved late in the process and answering the HTA agency's questions is not as effective as being involved from the start and assisting them in focusing the questions that are being asked. A HTA may be negative or positive depending on the outcome but only by involvement in the process can you influence the decisions taken. If the HTA result is negative then being involved can then lobby the government and point out the flaws in the decision with the knowledge of how the decision was made.

As this process is relatively new and more and more countries are using these methods, it is important to take a proactive approach to this process.

- Start now with learning the methods used in other countries to do a HTA. Within the patient organisation appoint one or more people with an interest and encourage them to develop their knowledge

- Find out about your National HTA agency and what HTA's they have planned
- Every country has a different approach and preference for different methods. Learn about the approach and the background to the methods they are using
- If you are asked to be involved in the process, get involved if you have the resources. If resources are unavailable look to other organisations that have been thorough the experience. Use the same people and build up knowledge now. This is a complicated process with specific terminology. A token representative or representation will not help in this process.
- If the HTA process does not ask for patient involvement, contact the agency carrying out the assessment and offer your help. People who might be affected by the assessment have an important perspective to provide. You should explain the experience you have (with the clinical situation and/or the technology) and the relevance of what you are able to contribute. If necessary lobby for involvement.
- Do NOT wait to be contacted by the HTA agency if a HTA on haemophilia will take place in your country. Contact them and politely but firmly insist that the views of your National haemophilia patient organisation must be considered by the HTA panel or otherwise you will view the process as fundamentally flawed.

6.1. Providing patient evidence

Along with having the right patient and the patient organisation collecting the information necessary it is also important to put all the documentation that the patient organisation will provide together in a comprehensive report for the HTA agency. They will separately have gathered the evidence based data from journals and publications and with the assistance of the clinicians and the pharmaceutical companies who provide the therapy. The report from the patient organisation needs to be planned clearly and concisely. The report should contain items such as:

a) Why your contribution is valid

   - Experience of an individual and the organisation submitting the evidence
   - Who the organisation represents
   - Services the organisation provides
   - Focus groups and surveys undertaken, statistical analysis from your own country and then outside the country.

b) A Commentary on existing data

   - Clinical trials – Positives and Negatives
   - Comparison of Methods
   - Provide a perspective on the well known evidence based data

c) Experience of the illness

   - Symptoms – A description of a bleed, quotes on the impact of pain associated with bleeds.

- How it affects daily living – Arthritis, Pain, work, etc.
- Short and long term impact on length and quality of life- HIV, Hepatitis C, vCJD risk
- Psychological and sociological effects of the illness and joint deformities due to bleeds

d) The impact of the treatment

- Benefits of the treatment – Prophylaxis, Home Treatment
- Impact on everyday life – School/Work, Pain, Exercise, Health state
- The psychological and sociological effects of the treatment and of not having access to the treatment
- Comparison's of countries with more/less access to treatment
- The financial impact of lack of treatment

6.2. *Working in partnership*

In a HTA process, patients are not the only group that have a legitimate interest in the results of an assessment. Insurance companies, scientific societies, clinicians, hospitals and industry will all have their own interests and some of them will be shared interests with the patients. Ideally, the key haemophilia clinicians in the country will co-operate and submit an agreed report and data to satisfy the requirements for evidence based data [1]. The haemophilia patient organisation should liaise closely with the clinicians. The organisation should be appraised of the evidence based data which is being submitted and should familiarise themselves with the key arguments and data. The organisation should co-operate with the clinicians in studies, surveys or data collection designed to strengthen the case being made. They should also share with the clinicians the experiential data they plan to submit. The highest possible degree of co-operation and co-ordination between the clinicians and the patient organisation are desirable to optimise the probability of a positive outcome from the process.

The patient organisation should also use the extensive network of the World Federation of Hemophilia (WFH) and the European Haemophilia Consortium (EHC) to provide them with additional data, resources or argumentation. Contact should be made with any other haemophilia societies who have gone through this process. Contact should definitely be made with other organisations in your country that have gone through this process. They can be an invaluable source of feedback and advice on how to approach the process and the HTA panel in your own country.

7. Introduction to terminology

As mentioned previously, HTA's have very specific terminology. An important aspect in learning about HTA's, is understanding this terminology and hence using it effectively in everything from planning experiential data collection to reviewing of published papers to presenting information to the HTA panel. There are a number of terms which will be explained in the next section as they are discussed such as cost effectiveness, value, equity etc and also in the glossary at the end of the monograph. However, there are a couple of terms that are key in any discussion about HTA's. They appear time and time again and are the building blocks of almost all HTA's. These are QALY, Utility and Outcome.

7.1. *Quality-Adjusted Life Year (QALY)*

This is a measure of benefit of health care combining the impact on both expected length of life and quality of life. Basically this means, a year of active normal life gained as the result of a treatment is rated higher than a year of living with reduced quality (such as being in extreme pain or being in hospital). It is often measured in terms of the level of a person's ability to perform activities of daily living, their freedom from pain and mental disturbance. It is measured by patients, or observers with knowledge in the area, rating these various states in relation to the specific disease by giving them scores.

7.2. *Utility*

In an economic evaluation generally means a measure of the value individuals attach to different outcomes (usually health). These are often used in QALYs to compare the length of time spent in different health states. A Utility can also mean a patient's preferred outcome.

7.3. *Outcome*

This is a test or treatment that impacts on health of a patient. Some examples of outcomes are the number of patients who fully recover from an illness, the amount of weight that patients lose or the number of hospital admissions.

7.4. *Challenges*

The main challenges that patient organisations and health professionals working in haemophilia could be involved in addressing are:

1. **The limits to the clinical and outcomes data available.** For example, in relation to prophylaxis, there is just one published randomised study comparing prophylaxis with on-demand factor VIII therapy [3]. This study (the Manco-Johnson study published in the New England Journal of Medicine) was conducted in young boys aged under 30 months who were followed-up to the age of 6 years: 93% of boys in the prophylaxis group had normal joints compared to 55% of the on-demand treatment group. This study had good duration

of follow-up but was in limited patient numbers ($n = 65$ in total), so there is a need for additional clinical evidence and studies to provide essential data to improve the robustness of cost-effectiveness analyses. Trials designed with health economic objectives in mind (i.e. to collect quality of life and resource use/cost data) would be valuable.

2. **The lack of a standard approach to utility measurement for QALYs and limited availability of appropriate utility data relevant for haemophilia.** Further data is required on the quality of life, in particular utilities, associated with on-demand and prophylaxis treatment in children and adults with haemophilia A.
3. **Therapy such as prophylaxis in haemophilia confers obvious current benefits to the individual but also very large future benefits as the damaging consequences of repeated bleeding will generally be avoided.** Most economic evaluations discount the future benefits of current therapy too severely (discount rates), especially for conditions such as haemophilia. This inevitably leads to a higher estimate of cost of therapy. Health economic evaluations generally value future quality of life benefits for haemophilia patients at a lower rate than current benefits in the same way we might value future costs at a lower rate than current costs for other conditions. The selection of appropriate discount rates by HTA bodies for health economic evaluations seems to be fairly arbitrary and varies across countries.
4. **The importance for economic analyses in haemophilia to adopt a society perspective with all key values captured.** This may include an acceptance that any child may be born with a life long relatively expensive to treat medical condition but the individual or family should not suffer unduly because of this.
5. **Incorporating equity considerations.** A strong case can be made for expanding or weighting the QALY to bring particular equity considerations associated with haemophilia care (e.g. children affected, genetic disorder, rarity) into account?
6. **HTA bodies and decision makers can be reminded that haemophilia comes within the definition of an orphan disease and as such there are limits to the ability to conduct large studies in this field.** Also, specific groups such as those patients with inhibitors are even rarer. This should be taken into account by HTA bodies when considering the feasibility and uncertainty that is inherent in clinical and economic studies of orphan conditions. There is ongoing debate amongst health economists about the feasibility and validity of economic evaluation of orphan diseases.

In all the above areas (and other areas) there is scope for patient organizations and health professionals working in haemophilia to raise the level of debate with HTA bodies charged with estimating the cost-effectiveness of interventions for haemophilia patients.

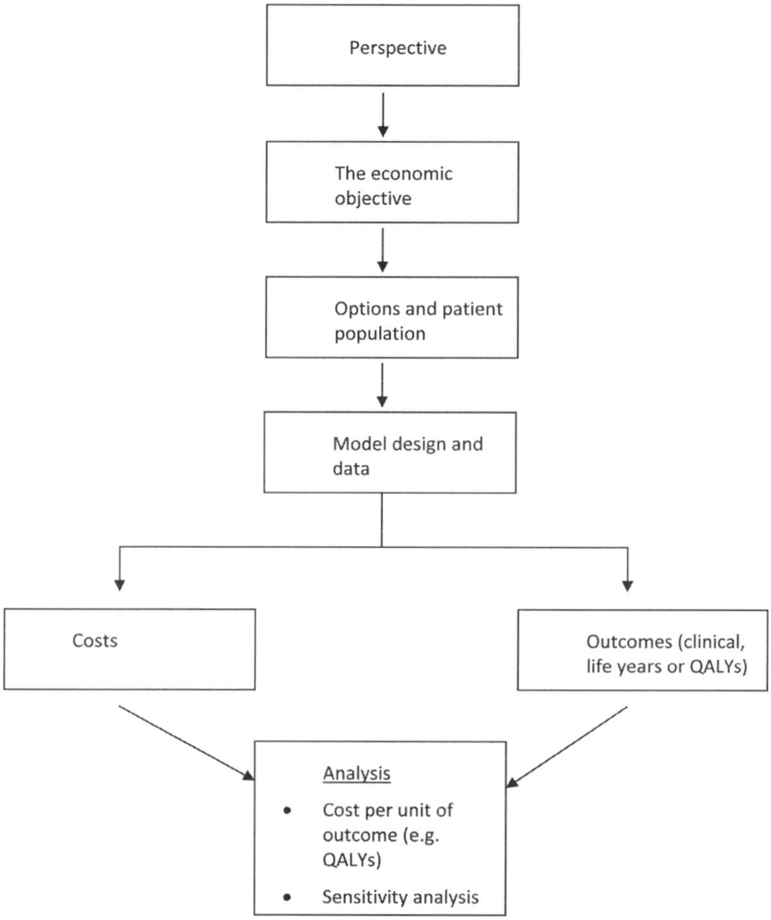

Fig. 1. The basic cost-effectiveness framework.

7.5. How is cost-effectiveness evaluated?

There is no one approach to performing cost-effectiveness analysis. A good example is the first box – perspective. As the perspective determines which values (for costs and benefits) are taken into account. The most common perspectives adopted are the healthcare payer, and the society perspectives. There are differences in approach between HTA agencies that use cost-effectiveness analysis for decision making purposes. For example:

– In the UK, NICE (covering England and Wales) and the Scottish Medicines Consortium (SMC) measure health effects using the concept of Quality Adjusted Life Years (QALYs). Both agencies assess costs from a health care payer

perspective when evaluating the cost-effectiveness of pharmaceuticals. The QALY measure focuses on the benefits to the patient and not, for instance, other family members/carers, A QALY weighting may be given to treatments that benefit patients at the end of life.
- In Sweden and The Netherlands, the TLV and NVTAG/CVZ, respectively, also adopt QALYs as the primary outcome measure, but unlike the UK and several other countries, the perspective of society is used for evaluating the cost-effectiveness of pharmaceuticals. Hence, costs and benefits to family members, carers and to the economy (e.g. economic productivity) are taken into account.
- In Germany, use of cost-effectiveness analysis by the national HTA agency (IQWIG) to support reimbursement decision making and guidance is still in the process of development but will not use the QALY. Instead they will involve the use of clinical outcome measures (e.g. bleeds avoided, surgery avoided) to compare health care technologies within a specific disease area.

Cost-effectiveness analyses in which the QALY is applied are called cost-utility analyses (CUA). The rationale behind the use of the QALY is that it is a generic measure of health benefit that can be applied to compare the cost-effectiveness of treatments across diseases. The QALY measure combines survival outcomes with a value (known as a utility) for the health related quality of life (HRQOL) associated with remaining life expectancy. Utility values have a special meaning in health economics. They represent individual's preferences for different states of HRQOL. They are measured on a scale of 0–1 with zero being equivalent to death (or worst possible health state) and one being perfect health. The scale of 0–1 is used as the aim is to use the utility score to calculate QALYs. Box A is an example of how a QALY is calculated and used to demonstrate cost-effectiveness.

Figure 2 provides an illustrative graphic of the 0–1 scale with examples of possible heath states (using the headache/migraine related example) corresponding to each score.

Box A: Calculating the QALY and cost-effectiveness

A haemophilia patient who has several bleeds per month may have a score of 0.5 (on the scale of 0–1) which is quite a poor quality of life. If they live for the next 10 years with this quality of life the QALYs they get are five (10×0.5). A treatment that could prevent bleeds could increase the quality of life score to close to normal (say 0.9). So, then they would get 9 QALYs (a gain of 4 QALYs).
The way we look at this is to work out the additional net costs and divide them by the additional benefits – the QALYs gained. So if over a 10 year period the extra net costs are €60,000 per patient for four extra QALYs gained then the cost per QALY gained would be €15,000.

How can we tell whether a treatment is cost-effective using the QALY approach? This depends on the value placed on each QALY gained in the country where the evaluation is being performed. In the UK, NICE and SMC use a benchmark of €23,000 to €34,000 per QALY gained. In Sweden, the benchmark used is closer to

1	PERFECT HEALTH
0.9	Normal health
0.8	Headache once a week
0.7	Migraine once a week
0.6	3 migraines per week
0.5	Daily migraines
0.4	Regular severe migraines
0.3	Regular severe migraines and other pain
0.2	Regular pain (including severe migraines)
0.1	Constant migraines and pain
0	DEATH

Fig. 2. Illustration of health states on the 0–1 scale.

€50,000, although it can vary based on factors such as the severity of the disease. In general, these benchmarks have been arbitrarily set but can be argued to reflect the willingness to pay of healthcare payers (in the UK) or society (in Sweden) for health benefits. The benchmark is higher in Sweden, which may be due to this greater focus on society values. Although the QALY approach has been adopted as the main measure for cost effectiveness, there are a few issues with the concept.

Key issues to consider in relation to QALY's, cost-effectiveness and haemophilia are

- Just how robust is the measurement of utilities and QALYs?
- Whose perspective is included when measuring costs and QALYs? Whose values count?
- What costs are included?
- How are health benefits/QALYs that occur in the future valued?
- How much uncertainty [in clinical effectiveness data] is acceptable?

The point was made earlier in the chapter that these values are subjective. Consideration should be given to also examining the data using measures such as the number of bleeds avoided annually or increased ability to work or attend school or college because of the therapy provided.

Table 1
The valuation of utilities

Valuation method	Description
Standard Gamble	Respondents are asked to specify the likelihood of accepting a gamble resulting in either perfect health (for life) or death, rather than experiencing a health state for certain for life (e.g. 5 bleeds per 3 months). For example, they might accept the gamble if there were a 60% probability of perfect health, so the utility for the bleed health state would be 0.6 (60% divided by 100%).
Time trade-off	Respondents are asked to specify the amount of time they would give up in perfect health to avoid a longer time with the health state in question (e.g. 5 bleeds per 3 months). For example, assuming a scenario of 10 years in the health state (followed by death), the individual might be willing to give up 4 years to be in perfect health (followed by death), so the utility for the health state would be 0.6 (6 years divided by 10 years).
Rating Scale (VAS)	Respondents are simply asked to place a mark for the health state on a visual analogue scale from 0–100, with 0 = death, 100 = perfect health. A utility of 0.6 for the 5 bleeds per 3 month health state means the respondent placed the mark at 60 on the scale (rescaled so that 60 = 0.6).

7.6. Measurement of health utilities

Utility measurement is the core of the QALY, but also the most controversial aspect. The basic method of utility measurement within a cost-effectiveness analysis consists of two main aspects:

a) A clear and accurate description of the key attributes of health states or outcomes that impact on health related quality of life.
b) Valuation of those health states/outcomes on the 0–1 utility scale.

8. There are two main approaches to the measurement of the utility: direct and generic measurement

Direct measurement consists of a set of methods by which utilities for disease and/or treatment specific health states and outcomes are directly valued by patients or members of the public. In contrast generic measurement consists of a variety of questionnaires that measures patient utility for general aspects of health such as level of mobility or level of anxiety, or ability to perform usual activities. Within each category there are a number of different techniques available none of which tend to produce the same results [7].

8.1. Direct measurement techniques for Utilities

The main direct measurement techniques used in health technology assessment are the standard gamble (SG), time trade-off (TTO) and rating scale (visual analogue scale). A short summary of each of these techniques is provided in Table 1. There is no correct method for carrying out these measurements. SG and TTO are better

Table 2
Comparison of three popular generic utility instruments

EQ 5D	SF 6D	HUI
5 health domains (mobility, self care, usual activities, pain/ discomfort, anxiety depression) Utilities based on TTO methods Valued by general population (in several countries) Only adult version currently validated Has a greater range of scores than SF 6D May lack sensitivity due to fewer domains especially in less severe health problems Quick questionnaire to complete Ceiling effects found (large percentage of respondents report no problem)	6 health domains (physical functioning, role limitation, social functioning, pain, mental health, vitality) Derived from the validated generic quality of life questionnaireSF36 Based on SG methods Valued by general population (in UK) Only adult version currently validated Floor effects found (large proportion of respondents report low scores)	7–8 health domains (HUI3) (speech, vision, ambulation, dexterity, emotion, cognition, pain) Based on SG methods Valued by general population (in Canada) Includes a version available for use in children (HUI2) Has stronger emphasis on sensory elements than other instruments

measures of preference but VAS has the advantage of simplicity. Each of these measures is completed by either patients with the condition or health state of interest, carers/parents or members of the public. There are some challenges with these methods such as accurate description of the health states. It is difficult to draw up descriptions that capture the key quality of life and other affects for the health states that would not be considered biased (i.e. exaggerating the impact) by HTA agencies and decision makers

8.2. Generic utility questionnaires

These are questionnaires that capture patient responses to questions relating to general aspects of health such as level of mobility or level of anxiety, or ability to perform usual activities. Overall, the instrument that is most popular with HTA agencies is the EQ-5D (also known as the EuroQol), but other instruments used include the Health Utilities Index (HUI) and SF 6D [8]. A short description and comparison of these instruments is provided in Table 2. They have different strengths and weaknesses for use with different disease areas – for example, the EQ 5D may be better used in severe conditions, whereas HUI may be better for sensory disabilities (e.g. impaired vision). Further details on the methods of utility measurement can be found in the monograph 'What are health utilities?' [9]

9. Cost-effectiveness analysis in haemophilia

In Europe, debates on the issue of HTA and health economic evaluations and the use for drug access decisions are increasing in frequency. Some of the questions in relation to Haemophilia that could be asked by HTA agencies over the next 5 years are:

- Is it cost-effective to provide prophylactic use of Factor VIII or Factor IX for severe Haemophilia or is on-demand treatment when bleeding actually occurs, a more cost-effective therapy?
- Is provision of prophylactic therapy for adults with severe Haemophilia cost effective?
- Are recombinant clotting product cost-effective compared to use of plasma derived products?
- Will new recombinant Factor VIII products which have an extended efficacy offer good value for money compared to existing recombinant products such that they should be reimbursed?
- Is prophylaxis for patients with inhibitors cost effective?

Question three is arguably the least likely to be addressed first in the developed world due to the history of HIV and Hepatitis in the past although it may come in time. The fourth question has not been relevant to date, but as new products come to market offering increased benefits such as less frequent infusion but at a potentially higher cost per unit it is going to be important that these are shown to be cost-effective. These may well be subjected to an Innovative HTA process specifically designed for new or novel therapies. Question five covers another area of growing cost and payer interest is the question of the cost-effectiveness of different products for the treatment of joint bleeds in haemophilia patients with inhibitors to factor VIII.

The first and second questions are those which are more likely to be examined earlier especially in relation to treatment of adults with primary prophylaxis. Therefore it is worth examining these in some detail

10. The Prophylaxis example

Prophylaxis is recognised as the optimal therapy for children with severe Haemophilia. This has been recognised from the results of the joint outcome study [3] which demonstrated that prophylaxis in children was associated with an 83% reduction in joint damage. Prophylaxis has been widely used in Sweden for many years as the preferred therapy for both children and adults. Prophylaxis from early childhood prevents many of the debilitating joint and muscle bleeds associated with on demand therapy. It may also play a role in reducing the risk of intracranial bleeding and in reducing the risk of inhibitor development (personal communication Dr. Günter Auerswald, Germany). It clearly enhances the quality of life [10]. Prophylaxis as optimal therapy for severe Haemophilia is one of the principles of Haemophilia care espoused by the European Association for Haemophilia and Allied Disorders. (EAHAD) [11]. These principles in turn have been endorsed by both the WFH and EHC. The European Division for the Quality of Medicines (EDQM) in their deliberations on optimal use further stated that prophylaxis in adults should also be considered [12]. Prophylaxis is widely used as the optimum therapy in many countries. In a survey of 19 European countries in 2009 [13], ten countries made prophylaxis available to all children with severe Haemophilia and a further four countries made prophylaxis available to 50–75% of children. The countries where prophylaxis was not available to children were those with very sub standard access to treatment and a low GDP per capita.

The majority of the published health economic studies have focused on comparing the costs and outcomes (bleeds and surgery/hospitalisation avoided) associated with the use of primary prophylaxis with factor VIII concentrate for severe haemophilia A with on-demand treatment (i.e. treat when the bleed occurs). These studies date back to the mid 90's, but it wasn't until 2002 that the first cost-utility analysis of primary prophylaxis with QALYs as the outcome measure was published [14]. The general conclusion from the studies is that primary prophylaxis is clinically superior (in terms of reducing bleeds and reducing need for surgery) and produces better health related quality of life outcomes compared to on-demand treatment of severe haemophilia A, but this comes at (significant) additional cost.

The cost-utility studies in prophylaxis have used similar health economic modelling approaches but come up with remarkably different results. There have been at least 5 such studies published showing the estimated QALY estimates of FVIII prophylaxis in Haemophilia. A.:

Study	Cost per QALY estimate (US $)
Miner 2009	50,000
Miner 2002	65,000
Roosendahl 2007	300,000
Risebrough 2008	420,000
Lippert 2005	1.2 m–2.7 m

It is worth examining the different QALY cost estimates for prophylaxis with these studies and the reasons why the cost per QALY varies to such a large extent. Some of the reasons may include:

- The time period of the study.
- The assumed number of bleeding episodes annually with on-demand therapy
- The assumed cost per unit of the factor concentrate
- The discount rate applied to the future benefits of current therapy.

Typically, HTA agencies heavily discount the future benefits of current therapy. However prophylaxis in Haemophilia has current benefits for the individual but also very real and significant future benefits. These should not be discounted heavily by the process. A child being treated with prophylaxis will derive great benefit during his adult life from his childhood treatment as he should be able to avoid joint and muscle damage, gain a good education, employment and live a normal lifespan with a near normal quality of life.

Clearly, it would be difficult to make a strong case for prophylaxis in adults if the Incremental Cost (ICER) per QALY was in excess of US$ 2 million as in the Lippert study [15]. There are a number of possible reasons why this figure may be so high. This paper examined a short time period of only 1 year for the analysis which is too short to take into account long term outcomes. The difference in the quality of life measured with on demand therapy (0.7427) compared to prophylaxis (0.7754) was extremely low. This small difference means that the additional cost appears remarkably high.

To demonstrate how we arrive at the Incremental Cost per QALY, using the Lippert study as an example:

> A **Utility value** (**QALY**) of a person under 30 with on-demand Treatment (HIV negative) is **0.7427** and costs €85,451
>
> A **Utility value** (**QALY**) of a person under 30 on Prophylaxis (HIV negative) is **0.7754** and costs €157,972
>
> The difference in cost is€72,521 for 0.0328 of a QALY (0.7754–0.7427)
>
> The Incremental Cost of a full QALY (€72,521 divided by 0.0328): €2,212,749

If however we look at the same data and look at the cost per bleed avoided:

A person under 30 with on-demand Treatment has an average of 16.7 bleeds a year at a cost of €85,451 A person under 30 on prophylaxis has an average of 5.9 bleeds a year at a cost of €157,972. The difference in cost is €72,521 but by using prophylaxis, the individual avoids 10.8 bleeding episodes. The cost per bleeding episode avoided is € 6,653. This is a much lower and more comprehensible figure. The impact of a single bleed can be devastating if it is, for example, a central nervous system or other life threatening bleed. It can be life altering if it is limb threatening. At the very least, it will cause acute pain, loss of short term function and possibly add to the long term joint or muscle damage which may limit the ability of the individual to fully participate in society. This is without considering the disruption and anxiety caused to the individual, their family or carer and the impact on their education and employment.

In Canada, the Riseborough study [16] showed a cost per QALY for primary prophylaxis versus on-demand treatment for children aged up to 6 years of over $500,000 Canadian (€320,000). In this study, Prophylaxis was associated with a utility (QALY) value of 0.95 and on demand with a surprisingly high value of 0.875.

The 2009 update study [6] by Miners et al., (updating an economic analysis published in 2002) shows a base case cost per QALY gained for lifelong primary prophylaxis of £37,000 (€41,000), which has improved from the initial 2002 estimate of £46,500 (€51,000) [14]. This is still above the usual threshold approved by NICE in the UK of £30,000 but is not excessively so. This study discounts the future benefits of current prophylactic therapy to a lesser extent. In addition the utility (QALY value)

Table 3
Utility estimates for prophylaxis and on-demand treatment from three published studies

Study	Utility for on demand health state (mean)	Utility for prophylaxis health state (mean)	Incremental cost per QALY gained prophylaxis vs. on-demand (converted to Euros)
Miners et al.,[23] 2009 (UK)	0.66	0.87	51,000
Risebrough et al.,[22] 2008 (Canada)	0.87	0.95	320,000
Lippert et Al	0.7427	0.7754	875,000–1,970,000

associated with prophylaxis in a 30 year old (0.87) showed a greater difference when compared with on-demand therapy (0.66) that that seen in the Lippert study [15]. This larger difference translates into a much lower incremental cost per QALY of US $50,000.

The differences in the utility values seen with the Miners study seem to the authors to be more realistic and they certainly correspond to a far greater extent with the results of the study undertaken on the different outcomes of prophylactic therapy versus on demand therapy in young adults in Sweden, Ireland, UK and France [17]. This study found an average utility value on prophylaxis of 0.93 when compared to 0.73–0.76 for on demand therapy. The treatment costs were not examined in this case so the ICER per QALY could not be calculated. However we would expect it to be much closer to the figure seen in the Miners study that that seen in the Riseborough or Lippert studies.

There is reason for hope (given also other arguments relating to equity and other special circumstances of haemophilia care) that primary prophylaxis would not be instantly dismissed as cost-ineffective by HTA bodies such as NICE. However, if future health economic analyses were to produce results similar to those in the Canadian or Lippert studies this would give less cause for optimism. It is likely that HTA agencies will use similar approaches to the economic modelling as has been used in the UK [14] and Canadian [16] studies.

Recently, as mentioned above, the Irish Haemophilia Society in conjunction with the Swedish, UK, and French societies collected experiential data and compared prophylaxis, on-demand or combined treatment in 20–35 year old males with severe haemophilia [17]. Medical and psychological data were collected from 58 males (average age 27.5 $\pm$ 4.7 years) in a phone survey. As part of this survey an EQ-5D questionnaire was filled out. This asks 5 broad questions and the utility values are then read from a chart. Values range from 0 (death) to 1 (perfect health) The survey demonstrated that people with severe haemophilia in Sweden in this age group spent a significantly higher percentage of their life on prophylaxis, reported lower presence of target joints, less major bleeds and significantly lower mobility problems. On a scale of 0–1, the EQ-5D showed respondents from Sweden with an average utility of 0.93 having a better quality of life compared to Ireland (0.76), UK (0.73) or France (0.73). Respondents on prophylaxis reported lower average bleeds per year (Mean 3) compared to on-demand treatment (Mean 26) or on-demand with intermittent periods on prophylaxis treatment (Mean 20). They also reported lower presence of target joints and significantly lower mobility problems based on the EQ5D. On demand treatment was associated with more days missed at work (Mean 33 days) compared to those on prophylaxis (Mean 3 days.) or on combined treatment (Mean 11 days). Sixteen people reported having no target joints with 15 of these living in Sweden. Prophylaxis started at an early age and continued into adulthood results in less bleeding, less damage to joints and less time missed at work. Prophylaxis increases mobility and the ability to do everyday activities and improves the health related quality of life of people with severe haemophilia. This type of information from an experiential point of view is vital for societies to collect. This is information that can be put in the report or submission from the patient organisations and then discussed with the HTA panel.

The perceived additional cost of prophylaxis may appear high when compared to other HTAs which have been carried out. In Ireland, the ICER per QALY of introduction of Human Pappiloma Virus vaccination for girls was estimated at €17,383. The ICER for the use of statins has been estimated at between €17,000 and €33,800 The ICER cost of prophylaxis from the published studies varies from €36,000–€304,000. This seems untenable but it should be remembered that the single greatest effect of the provision of suboptimal and unsafe Haemophilia treatment in the past four decades was the infection of thousands of people with haemophilia with HIV, Hepatitis A, B and C. Perhaps a more realistic comparator therefore would be to compare the incremental cost of prophylaxis, not to provision of statins, but to blood safety measures. Health authorities will agree to higher incremental costs for blood safety measures which prevent transmission of blood borne viruses. If a new blood borne virus is transmitted, people with Haemophilia will once again find themselves at risk or at worst in the eye of the storm. Incremental costs per QALY for blood safety measures which have been approved vary from €300,000 to €47 million. (data collected by Health Information and Quality Agency,Ireland). For example, the ICER per QALY for NAT testing of Whole Blood Donations for HIV, Hep B or Hep C was $4.3–$9.1 million [18]. The ICER for Hepatitis B testing for post transfusion Hepatitis B using NAT testing versus an Enhanced Sensitivity HBsAG assay was €47 million [19].

In this context the economic cost of providing prophylaxis for persons with severe haemophilia is very cost effective.

11. Comparative Effectiveness Research (CER)

The cost of health care in the U.S.A. has, for many years, been a topic that has energized legislators and policy makers. The Congressional Budget office in 2007 stated that "only a *limited amount of evidence is available* about which treatments work best for which patients and whether the added benefits of more-effective but more-expensive services are sufficient to warrant their added costs – yet current practice tends to adopt more-expensive treatments *even in the absence of rigorous assessments* of their impacts" [16].

HTA is not widely used in the U.S.A., where an alternative system called comparative effectiveness research (CER) is used. CER is the direct comparison of existing healthcare interventions to determine which work best for which patients and which pose the greatest benefits and risks. The core question of comparative effectiveness research is which treatment works best, for whom, and under what circumstances. Unlike HTAs, CER focuses on the effectiveness of interventions and not on the cost-effectiveness.

The Institute of Medicine (IOM) committee has defined CER as "the generation and synthesis of evidence that compares the benefits and harms of alternative methods to prevent, diagnose, treat, and monitor a clinical condition or to improve the delivery of care. The purpose of CER is to assist consumers, clinicians, purchasers, and policy makers to make informed decisions that will improve health care at both the individual and population levels." CER involves the conduct of systematic and structured reviews of the existing evidence for the efficacy, clinical benefits and/or safety of drugs, diagnostic tests, other healthcare technologies, different service plans and structures, or the generation of new evidence on comparative effectiveness of interventions or services.

CER is an important component of President Obama's healthcare reforms, and was signed into law as part of the American Recovery and Reinvestment Act (ARRA) in February, 2009. A total of $1.1 billion of government funds have been allocated for CER, to "inform healthcare decisions by providing evidence on the effectiveness, benefits, and harms of different treatment options" [17]. A new council, the Federal Co-ordinating Council for Comparative Effectiveness Research, has been set up to coordinate research and guide investments in comparative effectiveness research funded by the Recovery Act.

The new U.S. Health reform bill (Section 6301) establishes a private, nonprofit entity (the Patient-Centered Outcomes Research Institute) governed by a public-private sector board appointed by the Comptroller General to identify priorities provide for the conduct of comparative outcomes research. It requires the IOM to ensure that subpopulations are appropriately accounted for in research designs. It prohibits any findings to be construed as mandates on practice guidelines or coverage decisions and contains patient safeguards to protect against discriminatory coverage decisions by the department of Health and Human Services (HHS) based on age, disability, terminal illness, or an individual's quality of life preference. The act provides funding for the IOM and authorizes and provides funding for the Agency for Health Research and Quality to disseminate its research findings (as well as other government-funded research), to train researchers in comparative research methods, and to build data capacity for comparative effectiveness research.

Depending on the results of the research recommendations, changes to individual patient treatment plans could be made. In 2009, the U.S. Institute of Medicine identified 100 priority study topics for CER relating to a range of diseases, service delivery options, and disability and health inequalities [18]. More than half the topics related to service delivery. Prominent disease areas included cardiovascular disease, geriatrics, mental health, and pediatrics. Interestingly for hemophilia, the IOM recommended CER be conducted on rare diseases that disproportionately affect certain subgroups of the population. Absent from CER is any notion of using health economics to assess the cost-effectiveness of different interventions. In a healthcare policy sense, cost-effectiveness remains a largely taboo term in the U.S.

The first research grants for CER are starting to be awarded. For example, the U.S. Society of Nuclear Medicine (SNM) has been awarded US $48,000 to hold a conference to develop research on the comparative effectiveness of position emission topography relative to other molecular imaging techniques, primarily for the diagnosis and management of cancer [19]. As yet, specific hemophilia research has not been funded for CER, but as a rare and expensive treatment area, it could well attract attention.

The sort of research advocated using CER would not be considered novel in Europe. HTA involving systematic reviews of clinical effectiveness to inform policy decisions has been standard in many European countries for several years. However, as it is government-led research, it represents a cultural shift for the U.S. Critics argue that CER findings could lead to direct rationing, government intrusion into the doctor-patient relationship, and could halt progress in 'personalized medicine' that is growing in popularity in the U.S. There is a concern that the main rationale for CER is to contain cost, rather than to improve service and access to treatment. If it is just about costs and coverage restriction, then hemophilia treatments could suffer under CER implementation. If it does what it is meant to do, then it could help improvement in healthcare quality and outcomes, including those for hemophilia patients.

Anyone is allowed to make suggestions for research topics for CER, so there are opportunities for hemophilia societies to take direct action and suggest research that would be most useful for patients.

12. Conclusions

HTA is likely to become an increasingly important influence in decisions about what is provided in healthcare, whether screening for diseases or treatments for serious illnesses. Already in Europe there is considerable discussion about greater collaboration between HTA agencies. It is important that HTA takes account of the needs of the people who will be most affected by its recommendations: patients, their caregivers and the public.

As a key component of health economic evaluations the QALY concept can be criticised in terms of limits to what it captures as a measure of benefit. Although QALYs are a measure of value of health and health related quality of life, they may not capture all the key outcomes for specific patients such those with haemophilia. The great variety of techniques and generic instruments available for utility measurement is a concern as the results they produce vary and there is not a clear way of justifying which is the most valid method to use in each circumstance.

For the time being QALYs are here to stay and are being used by HTA agencies around the globe to appraise new health technologies for their cost-effectiveness. It is expected the haemophilia treatment and care will be subject to this scrutiny across countries with the expectation that decisions on resource allocation and reimbursement will follow.

So whilst arguments can be raised against QALYs it is important for now for patient organisations and health professionals work with the QALY paradigm by understanding the methods, limitations and opportunities of them within health economic analyses in haemophilia. Going forward it would be useful if patient organisations were to join forces with sympathetic health economists and clinicians to design studies to fill the key data limitations (especially around utilities), and to lobby HTA agencies on the importance of a taking a broad perspective on costs and outcomes (including values of the parent/carer as well as the patient and society).

While participating in a HTA can be time consuming and challenging, it is a real opportunity to influence the delivery of healthcare. Patient and public input can help determine whether a new treatment is made available.

The challenges faced by the Haemophilia community due to economic constraints will increase in the future [20]. All the key stakeholders- patient organisations, clinicians and industry must respond and should, when appropriate, co-operate. Pharmaceutical companies should ensure that competition between them does not lead to damaging messages being delivered to HTA agencies which could serve to deprive people with haemophilia of the required therapy. Clinicians in each country should optimise their co-operation with each other and co-ordinate their submission of key clinical data. Clinicians should also ensure that they have a close working relationship with the national haemophilia patient organisation. Collaboration on the collection of evidence based and Experiental data should be a key goal [21]. The patient organisation in each country should be fully aware of the economic realities and pressure points on their health care budgets nationally. They should work in co-operation with clinicians and with other national patient organisations to collect the data required to vigorously defend or improve their access to care and treatment. They should have knowledge of and clearly understand the key evidence based data which supports optimum treatment and equally understand the data which could be used to advocate for a reduced standard of care. They should proactively collect Experiental data on an ongoing basis. Once a HTA is announced, it may be too late to collect the data at that point in time to influence the process. They should seek to be involved in the process and formally consulted as early in the process as possible. Finally, and most importantly, they must not ignore these challenges and continue in the expectation that they will never have to confront these issues at any level. A HTA in Haemophilia in your country may not occur but knowledge of the economics of haemophilia has never been more important.

Appendix 1: List of HTA Agencies

Argentina	Institute for Clinical Effectiveness and Health Policy Tel: +54 11 4966 0082 E-mail: info@iecs.org.ar
Australia	Australian Safety and Efficacy Register of New Interventional Procedures – Surgical Tel: +61 8 8363 7513 E-mail: asernips@surgeons.org Adelaide Health Technology Assessment Tel: +61 8 8303 3575 E-mail: tracy.merlin@adelaide.edu.au Medical Services Advisory Committee Tel: +61 2 62896811 E-mail: msac.secretariat@health.gov.au
Austria	Ludwig Boltzman Institute of Health Technology Assessment, LBI@HTA (former ITA) Tel: +43(0)1-2368119-0 E-mail: office@hta.lbg.ac.at Gesundheit Österreich GmbH, Austrian Health Institute Tel.: +43 1 515 61-0 E-mail: info@goeg.at Hauptverband der Österreichischen Sozialversicherungsträger Tel:+43 (1) 711 32 E-mail:posteingang.allgemein@hvb.sozvers.at
Belgium	KCE – Belgian Health Care Knowledge Centre Tel: +32 2 287 33 88 or +32 2 287 33 97 E-mail: info@kce.fgov.be
Brazil	Tecnologia e Insumos Estratégicos, Departamento de Ciência e Tecnologia Tel: +55 61 3315 3197 E-mail: flavia.elias@saude.gov.br
Canada	Institute of Health Economics University of Alberta, Public Tel: +1 780 4484881 E-mail: ejonsson@ihe.ca Agence d'Évaluation des Technologies et des Modes d'Intervention en Santé Tel: +1 514 8732563 E-mail: Reiner.Banken@aetmis.gouv.qc.ca Canadian Agency for Drugs and Technologies in Health Tel: +1 613 226 2553 E-mail: tammyc@cadth.ca Ontario Ministry of Health and Long Term Care Tel: +1 416 314 3999 E-mail: MASinfo.moh@ontario.ca
Chile	Department of Quality and Patient Safety of the Ministry Health of Chile Health Technology Assesssment Unit Tel: +56 2 574 0567 E-mail:pkraemer@minsal.cl
Denmark	CAST – Center for Anvendt Sundhedstjenesteforskning og Teknologivurdering, University of Southern Denmark, Center for Applied Research and Technology Assessment Phone: +45 6550 1000 E-mail: sdu@sdu.dk DSI – Danish Institute for Health Services Research Tel.: 35 29 84 00 E-mail: dsi@dsi.dk DACEHTA – Danish Centre for Evaluation and HTA Tel: +45 72 22 74 00 E-mail: sst@sst.dk HTA and Health Service Research, Center of Public Health Tel: 8728 4750 E-mail: mtv-stf@rm.dk
England & Wales	NICE – National Institute for Health and Clinical Excellence Tel: +44 (0)845 003 7780 E-mail: nice@nice.org.uk National Institute for Health Research HTA Programme Tel: 023 8059 5586 E-mail: hta@hta.ac.uk

Estonia	University of Tartu, Department of Public Health Tel: +372 737 5100 E-mail: info@ut.ee
Finland	FinOHTA – Finnish Office for HTA Tel. +358 9 3967 2297 E-mail: finohta@stakes.fi
France	HAS – Haute Autorité de santé / French National Authority for Health Tel.: 01 55 93 70 00 CEDIT – Committee for Evaluation and Diffusion of Innovative Technologies, Direction de la Politique Médicale Tel: (33) 1 40 27 18 90 E-mail: info.cedit@sap.aphp.fr
Germany	DAHTA@DIMDI – German Agency for HTA at the German Institute for Medical Documentation and Information Tel: +49 221 4724-1 IQWIG – Institute for Quality and Efficiency in Health Care Tel: +49 (0)221 - 35685 – 0 German HTA Association Tel (0421) 218-3784
Hungary	HunHTA – Unit of Health Economics and Health Technology Assessment Tel: 0036-1-482-5147 E-mail: laszlo.gulacsi@uni-corvinus.hu
Ireland	HIQA – Health Information and Quality Authority Tel: +353 21 425 0610 E-mail: info@hiqa.ie
Israel	Israel Center for Technology Assessment in Health Care Tel: +972 3 530 3278 E-mail: ninaH@gertner.health.gov.il
Italy	ASR – Agenzia Sanitaria Regionale, Emilia Romagna E-mail: fsarti@regione.emilia-romagna.it Università Cattolica del Sacro Cuore, Policlinico universitario "A.Gemelli", Health Technology Assessment Unit and Laboratory of Health Economics (Institute of Hygiene) Tel. +39 06 3015 1 E-mail: rettorato@rm.unicatt.it
Korea	Committee for New Health Technology Aseessment Tel: +82 31 543 2636 E-mail: omy@cha.ac.kr
Latvia	VSMTA – Health Statistics and Medical Technology State Agency Tel: +371 67501590 E-mail: agentura@vsmtva.gov.lv
Lithuania	State Health Care Accreditation Agency under the Ministry of Health of the Republic of Lithuania Tel: +(370) 5 261 51 77 E-mail: vaspvt@vaspvt.gov.lt
Malaysia	Health Technology Assessment Section, Ministry of Health Malaysia Tel: +603 888 312 29 E-mail: htamalaysia@moh.gov.my
Mexico	Centro Nacional de Excelencia Tecnológica en Salud Tel: +52 55 5208 3939 E-mail: evaluacion@salud.gob.mx
Netherlands	CVZ – College voor zorgverzekeringen Tel: (020) 797 8555

New Zealand	Health Services Assessment Collaboration Tel: +64 3 345 8147 E-mail: hsac@canterbury.ac.nz
Norway	Norwegian Knowledge Centre for the Health Services Tel: +47 23 25 50 00 E-mail: Gro.Jamtvedt@kunnskapssenteret.no
Poland	Agency for HTA in Poland, AHTAPol Tel. +48 22 566 72 00 E-mail: szkolenia@aotm.gov.pl CEESTAHC – Central and Eastern European Society for Technology Assessment in Health Care Tel. +48 (0) 12 357 76 34 E-mail: sekretariat@ceestahc.org
Scotland	SMC – Scottish Medicines Consortium Tel: +44 141 225 5552 E-mail: smcsecretariat@nhshealthquality.org NHS Quality Improvement Scotland Tel: 0131 623 4300
Slovenia	Institute of Public Health of the Republic of Slovenia Tel. +386 (1) 2441 518 E-mail: knjiznica@ivz-rs.si
Spain	AETS – Agencia de Evaluación de Tecnologias Sanitarias Tel: + (34) 91 822 20 04; E-mail: aets@isciii.es AETSA – Andalusian Agency for Health Technology Assessment Tel: +34 955006638; E-mail: aetsa.csalud@juntadeandalucia.es CAHTA – Catalan Agency for Health Technology Assessment and Research Tel. +34 935 513 888 E-mail: direccio@aatrm.catsalut.net Galician Agency for Health Technology Assessment Tel (0034) 981 542 737 OSTEBA – Basque Office for Health Technology Assessment (AP) Servicio Canario de la Salud Tel.: + 34 945 019250 E-mail: Osteba-san@ej-gv.es UETS – Unidad de Evaluación de Tecnologías Sanitarias, Agencia Laín Entralgo Tel: +34 913089480 E-mail: uets.ale@salud.madrid.org
Sweden	SBU – Swedish Council on Technology Assessment in Health Care Tel: 08-412 32 00 E-mail: info@sbu.se
Switzerland	SNHTA – Swiss Network for Health Technology Assessment Tel: +41 31 322 15 86 E-mail: info@snhta.ch
Taiwan	Center for Drug Evaluation Tel: +886 2 2322 4567 E-mail: wyshau265@cde.org.tw
Thailand	Health Intervenion and Technology Assessment Program Tel: +66 259 0459 E-mail: hatai.l@hitap.net
USA	Agency for Healthcare Research and Quality Tel: +1 301 427 1612 E-mail: elise.berliner@ahrq.hhs.gov VA Technology Assessment Program Tel: +1 857 3644469 E-mail: vatap@med.va.gov

Acknowledgements

Some of the concepts and Appendix 1 have been adapted or reprinted from Understanding Health Technology Assessment, published by Health Equality Europe (June 2008) and An Introduction to Economic Concepts in Haemophilia authored by Brian O'Mahony, Declan Noone and Keith Tolley and published by the World Federation of Hemophilia and the European Haemophilia Consortium in 2010. Available at www.wfh.org or www.ehc.eu.

References

[1] Treatment of Haemophilia A and B and von Willebrand disease – A systematic Review. SBU, Sweden, 2011. E. Berntorp et al., (to be published).
[2] C.A. Ludlam, P.M. Mannucci and W.G. Powderly, Addressing current challenges in haemophilia care: consensus recommendations of a European Interdisciplinary Working Group, *Haemophilia* **11**(5) (2005), 433–437.
[3] M.J. Manco-Johnson, T.C. Abshire, A.D. Shapiro, B. Riske, M.R. Hacker, R. Kilcoyne et al., Prophylaxis versus episodic treatment to prevent joint disease in boys with severe haemophilia, *N Engl J Med* **357**(6) (2007), 535–544.
[4] E. Berntorp, *Willingness to Pay Study in Swedish Taxpayers*, Symposium, WFH International Congress, Vancouver 2006.
[5] St. Schlenkrich, Ch.Schubert, Prophylactic treatment in an adult person with haemophilia- effectiveness and costs. Haemophilia, 2010.
[6] A. Miners, Revisiting the cost-effectiveness of primary prophylaxis with clotting factor for the treatment of severe haemophilia A, *Haemophilia* **15**(4) (2009), 881–887.
[7] R. Busse, *IQWiG Methods for Assessment of the Relation of Benefits to Costs in the German Statutory Health Care System*, Version 1.0. 2009.
[8] G.W. Torrance, W.H. Thomas and D.L. Sackett, A utility maximization model for evaluation of health care programs, *Health Serv Res* **7**(2) (1972), 118–133.
[9] K.H. Tolley, What are health utilities? What is series, Available from www.whatisseries.co.uk, Hayward Medical Communications, 2009.
[10] S. Royal et al., Quality of Life in Haemophilia, *Haemophilia* **8** (2002), 44–50.
[11] B.T. Colvin et al., European principles of haemophilia care, *Haemophilia* **14** (2008), 361–374.
[12] Optimal Clinical Use of Blood Components, Proceedings, *European Directorate for the Quality of Medicines and HealthCare* (April 2009). Paul-Ehrlich -Institut.
[13] B. O'Mahony, D. Noone, P.L.F. Giangrande and L. Prihodova, Haemophilia care in Europe: A survey of 19 countries, *Haemophilia* **17**(1)(2011), 35–40. DOI: 10.1111/j.1365-2516.2010.02362x.
[14] A.H. Miners, C.A. Sabin, K.H. Tolley and C.A. Lee, Cost-utility analysis of primary prophylaxis versus treatment on-demand for individuals with severe haemophilia, *Pharmacoeconomics* **20**(11) (2002), 759–774.
[15] B. Lippert, K. Berger, E. Berntorp, P. Giangrande, B.M. van den, W. Schramm, et al., Cost effectiveness of haemophilia treatment: a cross-national assessment, *Blood Coagul Fibrinolysis* **16**(7) (2005), 477–485.
[16] N. Risebrough, P. Oh, V. Blanchette, J. Curtin, J. Hitzler and B.M. Feldman, Cost-utility analysis of Canadian tailored prophylaxis, primary prophylaxis and on-demand therapy in young children with severe haemophilia A, *Haemophilia* **14**(4) (2008), 743–752.
[17] D. Noone, B. O'Mahony, L. Prihodova, A survey of the outcome of prophylaxis, on-demand or combined treatment in 20–35 year old men with severe haemophilia in 4 European countries, *Haemophilia* **17**(5)(2011), Pe842–e843. DOI: 10.1111/j.1365-2516.2011.02582.x.

[18] B.R. Jackson, M.P. Busch, S.L. Stramer and J.P. AuBuchon, The cost-effectiveness of NAT for HIV, HCV, and HBV in whole-blood donations, *Transfusion* **43**(6) (2003), 721–729.
[19] D.A. Marshall, S.H. Kleinman, J.B. Wong, J.P. AuBuchon, D.T. Grima, N.A. Kulin et al., Cost-effectiveness of nucleic acid test screening of volunteer blood donations for Bepatitis B, Hepatitis C and human immunodeficiency virus in the United States, *Vox Sang* **86**(1) (2004), 28–40.
[20] B. O'Mahony, Haemophilia Societies, Challenges and Developments, *WFH Haemophilia Organisation Development Monograph Series*, (Updated, accepted for publication).
[21] B. O'Mahony, *HTAs in Haemophilia*, Presentation at EHC International Conference, Vilnius, 2009.

Pharmaceuticals Policy and Law 13 (2011) 161–165
DOI 10.3233/PPL-2011-0321
IOS Press

HTAs and rare diseases: How to assess their cost-effectiveness

Ceri J. Phillips[a,*] Dyfrig A. Hughes[b]
[a] *Swansea Centre for Health Economics, College of Human and Health Sciences, Swansea University, Wales, UK*
[b] *Centre for Health Economics and Medicines Evaluation, Institute of Medical and Social Care Research, Bangor University, Bangor, Wales, UK*

1. Introduction

The assessment of pharmaceuticals has, in recent years, expanded beyond efficacy and safety to cover economic implications and other consequences. The incorporation of an economic perspective and an assessment of cost-effectiveness into the decision-making process as to what therapies can be made available have aroused much debate and discussion, which at times has been quite heated. Newspaper headlines of people having to remortgage their houses to pay for 'life-saving' therapies and media frenzy when 'effective' treatments are denied to desperate patients are becoming all too common occurrences. The emotive nature of such 'decisions' are intensified when considering rare conditions [3]. In rare diseases, the low number of patients makes therapies highly expensive, as they try to recapture research and development costs, and unlikely to meet the thresholds for cost-effectiveness of payment agencies [1, 2]. The appropriateness of conventional metrics for assessing efficiency has been challenged [4,5] while issues relating to whether therapies for rare diseases warrant special status within health technology assessments and whether the 'conventional' approaches and criteria used to assess effectiveness and efficiency should be extended to incorporate equity and social values remain equivocal [1,2,5].

2. The rationale for assessing cost-effectiveness

The techniques of economic evaluation have been used to address the fundamental economic problem, that while we all have unlimited wants and desires, we only

*Corresponding author: Ceri J. Phillips, Swansea Centre for Health Economics, College of Human and Health Sciences, Swansea University, Swansea SA2 8PP, Wales, UK. Tel.: +44 (0) 1792295729; E-mail: C.J.Phillips@swansea.ac.uk.

have limited resources (time, energy, expertise and money) at our disposal to satisfy them. This situation has become particularly evident in health care and has been compounded by factors such as the increasing expectations of the population in relation to what can actually be delivered by healthcare services, the continuing advancements in health technology and medical science and the increasing health needs and demands of an ageing population. At the individual level we are constantly making choices as to how we allocate our time, into which activities we channel our energies and on what we spend our available funds. In spending time on one activity or purchasing a certain commodity, means that period of time and those funds are not available for other activities and for other purchases. The same issues relate to the health system: which patients to treat, when and with what therapies? The use of limited healthcare funds to provide treatments and care for rare diseases would mean that those funds would not be available for treatments in other disease areas, and where, in all probability, greater benefits could be generated. Therefore, if the objective of healthcare systems is to maximise the health gains for its residents, and if the cost-effectiveness of therapies for all diseases are evaluated using a common approach, it is unlikely that many treatments for rare diseases would be approved. The question as to whether rare diseases should be treated differently in relation to cost-effectiveness, and therefore how, is a highly pertinent one [2] and one which this paper seeks to explore.

3. Costing and valuing treatments for rare diseases

Regulations exist to support the research and development of drugs for rare diseases. These vary – in terms of definitions of orphan and ultra-orphan drugs, the rationale for such support and in terms of the support mechanisms provided – across various jurisdictions [2], but tend to include "incentives to pharmaceutical companies include market exclusivity for 10 years, reduction of licensing fees, assistance with marketing applications, direct access to the centralized procedure for marketing authorization and provision of specific research grants" [1]. The legislation and regulations have enabled the development of such drugs to be profitable, but the use of such policies have led to claims that they have generated what might be termed excess profit, they are inflationary [6] and have led to an increase in the number of orphan diseases [2]. Further, the legitimate question has been posed as to whether society should invest its limited resources to subsidise the development of technologies when the value of health gain generated is less than the costs incurred [2], which is likely to be the case with the treatment of rare diseases.

This raises the equity issue as to whether outcomes from treatments for rare diseases should be valued differently from health outcomes generated elsewhere. The utilitarian approach to distributive justice would contend that every individual's health gain is valued equally and therefore dismiss such investment. However, there are situations where individuals' health gain is not valued equally. For example, the National Institute for Health and Clinical Excellence (NICE) give greater weighting to outcomes that occur in end-of life treatments [7] so that the incremental cost-effectiveness ratios for these treatments would be in line with current cost-effectiveness thresholds.

The underlying rationale for legislation relating to orphan drugs is that all patients should be able to access the same quality of treatment and care, which mirrors the rights-based approach to equity considerations. A recent qualitative study from Australia has highlighted the importance of giving all groups a 'chance' of being treated and of not removing 'hope' from high-cost patients [8] although, while this might afford treatments being made available for rare diseases, it does not necessarily favour rare diseases over more prevalent conditions in relation to resource allocation decisions [1].

The rule of rescue principle [9] emphasises that individuals with needs for highly specialised treatments should not be abandoned – especially under conditions of resource constraints [1] and gives weight to the view that society does differentiate between treatments in the value attached to individuals' health gain, and place a higher value on health benefits among people with worse lifetime health prospects [10]. This is dependent on the 'rules of fair cooperation', which implies that basic healthcare in a pluralistic democratic society is a fundamental right. However, this has been challenged as being incompatible with other equity principles and theories of justice [2], with the case for special status for treatments in rare diseases resting on the question as to whether the value of health gain to individuals should be different for an individual with a common disorder and an individual with a rare disorder [2]. The counter to this is to recognise that once basic equitable healthcare is viewed as adequate – reflected in indicators such as infant mortality and life expectancy – then principles of fair cooperation should apply [11].

The lack of consensus on the issue is evident in a report from the NICE Citizens' Council, which reported that:

"Just over half (16) of Council members thought that, with certain conditions, the NHS should consider paying premium prices for drugs to treat patients with very rare diseases. A further four people thought that the NHS should pay whatever premium price is required for drugs to treat patients with very rare diseases. Seven of us concluded that the NHS should not consider paying premium prices for drugs to treat patients with very rare diseases, but should decide whether or not to provide ultra orphan drugs using the same clinical and cost effectiveness appraisals as any other treatment" [12].

The only empirical study conducted to date, to determine whether there were grounds for ignoring cost-effectiveness considerations in the case of treatments for rare diseases was a survey conducted among a random sample of over 1500 Norwegians aged 40-67. The findings indicated that while there was strong support that "all individuals should have equal access to health care regardless of cost" and that "patients with rare diseases should have the right to treatment even if the treatment is more expensive," there was little evidence that a "societal preference for rarity exists if treatment of patients with rare diseases is at the expense of treatment of those with common disorders" [13].

4. Assessing cost-effectiveness of treatments for rare diseases

The question then revolves not on whether treatments for rare diseases should be excluded from cost-effectiveness assessments but rather how they should be treated within the assessment framework? The adoption of weighted QALYs as a possible way forward for assessing cost-effectiveness has been advocated [4] and reflects the policy direction taken with regard to end-of-life treatments [7]. It would be necessary for the evidence of the effectiveness (and safety) of treatments for rare diseases to be explicitly demonstrated, accompanied by other criteria that will help to inform the decision and justify the additional weighting given to QALY gains in assessing the relative cost-effectiveness of such treatments. For example, the All Wales Medicines Strategy Group (AWMSG) has made explicit the conditions that will inform the assessment of cost-effectiveness of ultra-orphan drugs [14]:

- The degree of severity of the disease as presently managed, in terms of quality of life and survival
- Whether the medicine can reverse, rather than stabilise the condition
- Whether the medicine may bridge a gap to a "definitive" therapy (e.g. gene therapy), and that this "definitive" therapy is currently in development
- The innovative nature of the medicine, where AWMSG will consider whether the medicine:
    - represents a significant improvement on existing therapy (e.g. the medicine is able to treat a condition where there was previously no effective treatment) and;
    - whether it can plausibly generate substantial health gains over existing treatments for the individual (e.g. > 1 QALY)

Further, the assessment agency (AWMSG) has stated that ultra-orphan medicines will be appraised on a case-by-case basis, and all patients receiving approved medicines should be entered into registries for recording prospective measures of clinical outcome [14].

These requirements would involve engagement by manufacturers and distributors with the relevant assessment agency to determine the specific criteria that would be used with regard to treatments for rare diseases, but also to ensure that the portfolio of evidence relating to clinical effectiveness, safety and patients groups is appropriate and available. It is not sufficient for them to assume that the classification of their therapies as treatments for rare diseases enables them to bypass the rigorous processes and procedures that have been established and applied to treatments for common health conditions. Every effort should be made to construct a clinical development programme that incorporates assessments of resource utilisation, burden of disease and quality of life to be placed alongside effectiveness and safety considerations within their evidence portfolios.

5. Conclusion

Treatments for rare diseases enjoy certain privileges in relation to licensing and marketing authorisation that enable them to be developed profitably. The question as to whether they should be given additional positive discrimination in their favour with regard to the assessment of cost-effectiveness remains a contentious issue that revolves around the valuation of health gain achieved by such treatments relative to the gains generated by treatments for common conditions. The only societal study has demonstrated that there was little support for premium prices for rarity. Therefore the onus is on manufacturers of treatments for rare diseases to demonstrate that their products generate important clinical benefits that can be placed alongside the conventional metrics for assessing cost-effectiveness to enable assessment agencies to gauge the extent to which treatments for rare diseases can be said to represent value for money.

References

[1] D.A. Hughes, B. Tunnage and S.T. Yeo, Drugs for exceptionally rare diseases: do they deserve special status for funding? *QJM* **98** (2005), 829–836.

[2] C. McCabe, K. Claxton and A. Tsuchiya, Orphan drugs and the NHS: should we value rarity? *BMJ* **331** (2005), 1016. doi: 10.1136/bmj.331.7523.1016.

[3] D.A. Hughes, Rationing of drugs for rare diseases, *Pharmacoeconomics* **24** (2006), 315–316.

[4] D.F. Moore, M. Ries, E.L. Forget and R. Schiffmann, Enzyme replacement therapy in orphan and ultra-orphan diseases: the limitations of standard economic metrics as exemplified by Fabry-Anderson disease, *Pharmacoeconomics* **25** (2007), 201–208.

[5] M.F. Drummond, D.A. Wilson, P. Kanavos, P. Ubel and J. Rovira, Assessing the economic challenges posed by orphan drugs, *International Journal of Technology Assessment in Health Care* **23** (2007), 36–42.

[6] R.E. Ferner and D.A. Hughes, The problem of orphan drugs, *BMJ* **341** (2010), c6456. doi: 10.1136/bmj.c6456.

[7] National Institute for Health and Clinical Excellence. Appraising life-extending, end of life treatments. Available at: http://www.nice.org.uk/media/E4A/79/SupplementaryAdviceTACEoL.pdf (accessed 18/06/2011).

[8] J. McKie, B. Shrimpton, J. Richardson and R. Hurworth, The monetary value of a life year: evidence from a qualitative study of treatment costs, *Health Econonomics*, doi: 10.1002/hec.1660.

[9] J. McKie and J. Richardson, The rule of rescue, *Social Science and Medicine* **56** (2003), 2407–2419.

[10] P. Dolan, R. Shaw, A. Tsuchiya and A. Williams, QALY maximisation and people's preferences: a methodological review of the literature, *Health Economics* **14** (2005), 197–208.

[11] M. Gross, Ethics, policy and rare genetic disorders: the case of Gaucher disease in Israel, *Theor Med Bioeth* **23** (2002), 151–171.

[12] NICE Citizens' Council, Ultra Orphan Drugs, http://www.nice.org.uk/niceMedia/pdf/boardmeeting/brdjan05item4.pdf (accessed 19/06/2011).

[13] A.S. Desser, D. Gyrd-Hansen, J.A. Olsen, S. Grepperud and I.S. Kristiansen, Societal views on orphan drugs: cross sectional survey of Norwegians aged 40 to 67, *BMJ* **341** (2010), c4715. doi: 10.1136/bmj.c4715.

[14] All Wales Medicines Strategy Group, AWMSG guidelines for appraising medicines. http://www.wales.nhs.uk/sites3/Documents/371/Guidelines%20for%20appraising%20medicines.pdf (accessed 19/06/2011).

2. Patient perspectives

Pharmaceuticals Policy and Law 13 (2011) 169–176
DOI 10.3233/PPL-2011-0335
IOS Press

Health Technology Assessment and patients' rights: Assess versus access?

François Houÿez*, Yann Le Cam, Fabrizia Bignami, Flaminia Macchia and François Faurisson
Eurordis, European Organisation for Rare Diseases, Paris, France

Patients' organisations call for an assessment of the clinical added value of orphan drugs at the time of the marketing authorisation evaluation. The European Commission has commissioned Ernst & Young to explore the feasibility of a new Committee at the European Medicines Agency[1].

A new drug candidate faces a number of hurdles on its journey to reach the patient. Regulators are the first, and right after are the Health Technology Agencies and payers. Things can turn sour, from a political point of view, when that second scenario happens, when the regulators say "yes this drug is safe and effective" and the payers say "Oh well but we won't reimburse it".

Regulators and health technology assessment experts have recently started to harmonise their respective methodologies to avoid some degree of redundancy and contradictions in their respective opinions. Patients are participating in the decision making at the European Medicines Agency, and work closely with some national regulatory agencies. More systematic involvement with health technology assessment agencies is only beginning. This paper illustrates some of the issues patients are discussing with health technology assessment bodies.

Keywords: Health technology assessment, patients' representatives, Quality-Adjusted Life Years, Health Services Accessibility

1. Can the public opinion adhere to regulatory agencies decisions?

In the patient population, the perception is often that reimbursement and availability decisions are **arbitrary** ones. Not mentioning the threshold per Quality Adjusted Life Years gained (QALY), adopted by National Institute for Clinical Excellence[2] (NICE): if this is an absolute threshold and decisions are not adapted to the context of rarity, patients will have more and more difficulties understanding different conclusions from different Agencies. One agency (benefit/risk evaluation) can conclude that the product can be authorised but another one can decide that the medicine is not worth the expense. **It is really creating a large confusion in the public**.

---

*Corresponding author: François Houÿez, Eurordis, Plateforme Maladies Rares, 96 rue Didot, 75014 Paris, France. Tel.: +331 56 53 52 18; Fax: +331 56 53 52 15; E-mail: francois.houyez@eurordis.org.

[1]European Commission call for Tenders. Creation of a mechanism for the exchange of knowledge between Member States and European authorities on the scientific assessment of the clinical added value for orphan medicines. http://ec.europa.eu/eahc/documents/health/tenders/2010/EN/EAHC_2010_05_contract_award_notice.pdf.

[2]Michael Drummond, Corinna Sorenson. Nasty or Nice? A Perspective on the Use of Health Technology Assessment in the United Kingdom. Value in Health Vol 12, Supplement 2. 2009.

1.1. An illustration of a confused family

Listening to a mother with two boys affected by a rare disease during a meeting organised by RadioOrg (the national rare diseases alliance in Belgium), the paradox of authorised products that are not reimbursed because considered not cost effective was striking. The mother reported her two sons were suffering from the same rare disease. When a new product was recently authorised, their doctor prescribed the same product to both, strictly in line with the labelling and the indication. For one brother the prescription was accepted and the product could be reimbursed, but not for the other brother, as he was declared to be "not likely to respond". If the likeliness to respond is only 20%, or 10% or even less, and the disease is life-threatening, most of European citizens would like to give a try and see if he or she can benefit and would be concerned if an agency would deny access.

How can a mother explain to a child that he will not be treated because society considers that the expense is worth for his brother but not for him? How can the brothers look at each other when one is treated and the other is not? And how can we explain to this family what the term "indicated for" means finally?

1.2. Discrimination between countries

Patients feel discriminated, within families, within and between countries. Eurordis conducted a series of surveys on the availability of authorised orphan drugs in Europe. Here[3] are some results from the last one we conducted in 2007 (Fig. 1) among the 22 orphan drugs firstly authorised since the adoption of the EU orphan drug regulation in 1999. If we consider the three products that were authorised in 2001 taken as an example, six years later they were available in 13, 22 and 25 states respectively, but not in 27. In a modern European Union, how can European citizens understand that access to new medicines is conditioned by nationality?

1.3. Treatment tourism

As a consequence, **patients do travel to save their life**. The judgment from the European Court of Justice, case Geraets-Smits & Peerbooms dated 12/07/2001 is highly informative. Mr. Peerbooms felt into a coma following a road accident in December 1996. He was taken in a hospital in the Netherlands and then was transferred in a vegetative state to the University Clinic in Innsbruck in Austria, in 1997, where he received special intensive therapy using neurostimulation. He came out this coma and left the Innsbruck clinic in June 1997. **In the Netherlands, reimbursement was refused** as his health fund had not decided to make this treatment

[3]Eurordis Survey on Price and Availability of Orphan Drugs, 2007. http://www.eurordis.org/IMG/pdf/2007ODsurvey-eurordis.pdf.

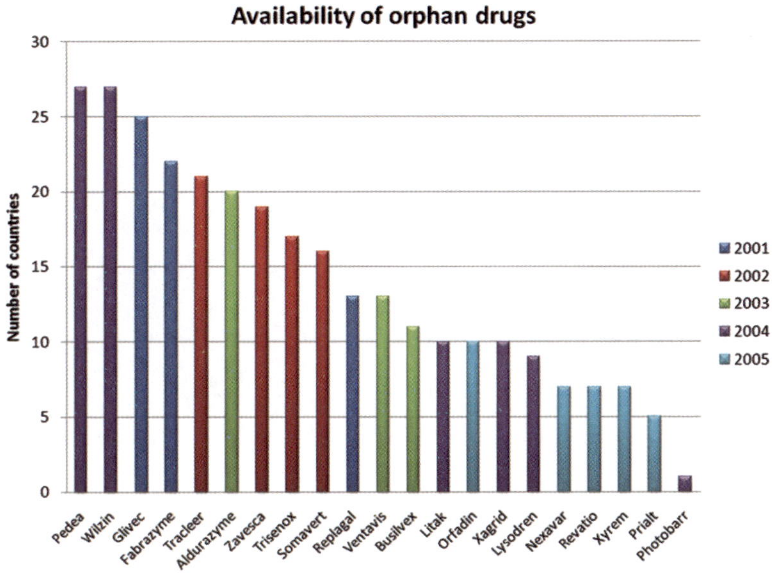

Fig. 1. Colours indicate the year of marketing authorisation. According to EU legislation, Member States have an obligation to respect a 180 days delay after marketing authorisation to conclude price and reimbursement negotiations with the marketing authorisation holder. Eurordis Price and Availability Survey 2007.

available to Dutch patients. He brought the case to the European Court of Justice that judged in his favour: the authorisation to purchase treatment **cannot be refused** where it appears that the treatment concerned is sufficiently **tried and tested by international medical science** (for example medicines evaluated by the European Medicines Agencies). The reimbursement can be refused only if **the same or equally effective treatment can be obtained without undue delay at an establishment having a contractual arrangement with the insured person's sickness insurance fund**.

At the end of 1996 in the United Kingdom, patients' representatives organised a press conference where they showed data from Aids hospitalisation rates decline in France whereas in the UK the National HealthCare Service was not even considering providing this product to the patients, but was still discussing how to best treat the opportunistic diseases, not the Human Immuno-deficiency Virus (HIV) infection itself.[4] Anti-HIV products that became largely available in France in April-May 1996 were still not largely available in the UK and the end of 1996. Still, these products can decrease HIV mortality by 90%, when the lethality of the infection was 100%. With such an efficacy, are cost-effectiveness studies really needed? In some

[4]Gilden D. Europeans eye new drug cocktails, *GMHC Treat Issues* **10**(12) (Dec 1996), 1–4.

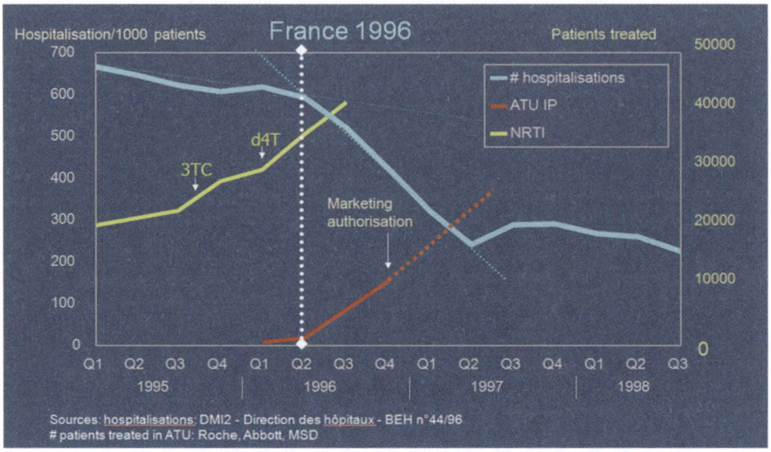

Fig. 2. Nucleoside Reverse Transcriptase Inhibitors (NRTI) became available via compassionate use programmes (ATU) between 1991 and 1995. HIV protease inhibitors (PI) became available via compassionate use programmes starting 1996. From the author.

countries health authorities were explaining to their patients that **first they need to assess properly the cost effectiveness before deciding to reimburse the product...**

2. Cost effectiveness studies can delay access, whereas compassionate use can accelerate it

Data from the French compassionate use scheme (Autorisation Temporaire d'Utilisation) show the number of HIV patients treated in the various compassionate use programmes and the hospitalisation rates for 1000 patients with HIV, in 1996 (Fig. 2). There were two declines in the hospitalisation rates: a slow one and a more rapid one, with an inflection point during second quarter 1996. First, one class of antiretroviral product was available, with different compassionate use programmes (3TC, d4T) and clinicians started to combine one or two antiretroviral products. Secondly, a more pronounced decline in hospitalisation rates was seen when a new class became also available, the protease inhibitors. In France, just two weeks after the initiation of the compassionate use, a decline in the hospitalisation rates could be measured as the immune system of the patients recovered quickly after the virus replication had been stopped.

Before the marketing authorisation (fall 1996), thousands of patients could benefit from this early acccss. Of course, the hospitalisation rates decline continued after the marketing authorisation. **Patients' organisations are highly interested in early access to promising drugs, and fear that even more complex discussion about HTA effectiveness will further delay access to drugs.**

2.1. When should HTA be assessed?

For promising new drugs for severe or life threatening diseases, the preferred scenario for patients is as follows:

1. Patients in the greatest need access the drug via a compassionate use programme
2. The product receives a marketing authorisation
3. All patients can access the drug when pricing and reimbursement decisions are made (the compassionate use programme lasts until the price and reimbursement decision are made)

In reality, the sequence is often:

1. The product receives a marketing authorisation
2. Health technology assessment starts, pricing and reimbursement decisions are made long time afterwards
3. And then large scale access, eventually

Considering that the 180 days legal delay[5] to decide on a price and on the reimbursement is rarely respected by member states, any HTA report that is requested after the marketing authorisation and that fails to conclude within 180 days is de facto not respecting European legislation.

So, when to ask for an HTA report?

Different approaches exist in the EU. In England for example, day 0 starts with the marketing authorisation, and then is followed by the NICE appraisal, which often lasts more than 300 days. If the product is cost effective then the NHS can provide it to the patients. Still there is another step: local hospitals need to decide to provide to its patients or not. For us, this is clearly **a budget containment orientated approach**.

In Germany, the Institute for Quality and Efficiency in Health Care (IQWIG) **has a different approach**:[6] firstly the marketing authorisation. From this moment, the product is purchased by health providers and patients can be treated. IQWIG appraisal can start and if the product is not considered cost effective, then the results of the assessment can be used to negotiate a price reduction until treatment/intervention becomes more cost effective, and **for us this is a more patients and public health orientated approach.**

2.2. QALYs are not adapted to rare and severe diseases

HTA assessment is used to prioritise different medical interventions and different patient populations who can benefit from them. In 1987 in Norway, a Commission

[5] Article 6(1) of Council Directive 89/105/EEC of 21 December 1988.

[6] IQWiG methods-a response to two critiques. J.J. Caro, E. Nord, U. Siebert, A. McGuire, M. McGregor, D. Henry, G. de Pouvourville, V. Atella and P. Kolominsky-Rabas, *Health Econ* **19**(10) (Oct 2010), 1137–1138.

defined principles that should be followed when prioritising interventions and patients, according to society's values. It concluded that severity of the disease is of primary importance, and that everyone should have a possibility to become as well as he or she can (to realise his/her health potential). These principles are not considered by the QALY method. NICE is aware of that limit, and NICE organised a citizens' workshop on how to introduce severity calculation of the QALY.[7]

QALYs do not quantify the value according to severity at baseline. To illustrate this, Erik Nord, senior adviser in the Norwegian Institute of Public Health (Fig. 3), has very elegantly showed that in the case of a patient who is disabled from birth (e.g. blind) with a health status of 0.6, and at the age of 40 suffers from a life-threatening disease (health status of being dead: 0): if he is successfully treated, he will eventually be cured but he will remain blind. His health gain will be 0.6 (his maximum health potential will be achieved). Comparing to a person who was not blind and who is treated for the same condition: this person will progress from 0 (risk of dying of the disease) to 1 (his maximum health potential will be achieved: disease cured and no blindness). The net gain is 0.6 for the disabled person and 1 for the non-disabled. Maximising QALYs always favour the wealthy against the disabled, and **we do not think that this is what the society wants to do, to always favour those who are wealthy compared to those who are not so wealthy, even if they can achieve most of their health potential**. Maximising QALYs do not reflect human society values.

3. Conclusions

EURORDIS has proposed[8, 9] to bring together all the knowledge and all the expertise that is known about a new orphan medicine at the time of marketing authorisation, and to come to an agreement between HTA agencies on which additional data are needed to complete the HTA report.

The proposal is to have a working party or a committee for the **common scientific assessment of the clinical added value of orphan drugs** (**CAVOD**). This proposal was accepted by the European Commission, the European Medicines Agency, and the industry (EBE and EFPIA.[10] If follows the recommendations of the Pharmaceutical

[7] Report on NICE Citizens Council meeting. Quality Adjusted Life Years (QALYs) and the severity of illness 31 January–2 February 2008. http://www.nice.org.uk/media/2C3/31/CCReportOnQALYsAndSeverity.pdf.

[8] See http://download.eurordis.org/europlan/3_EURORDIS_Guidance_Documents_for_the_National_Conference/7_Summary_CAVOD_%20Two_pages_29_October_2009.pdf.

[9] See full position paper: http://www.eurordis.org/IMG/pdf/Statement_Future_of_Orphan_Drugs_14_October_09.pdf.

[10] See EBE EuropaBio position: http://www.ebe-biopharma.org/index.php?option=com_news&task=view&id=188&Itemid=28.

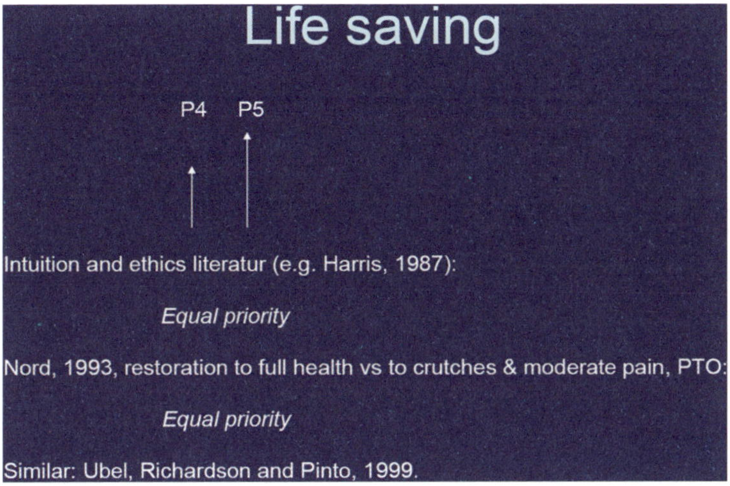

Fig. 3. Quality of Scale values and person trade-offs: QALYs always favour those who are wealthy. With permission, Erik Nord, Senior Adviser. Norwegian Institute of Public Health.

Forum.[11]

The rationale is that the European Medicines Agency already rigorously assesses the orphan drug: its significant benefit (orphan drug designation), its benefit/risk ratio and many other characteristics. **Sponsors of orphan drug designation are already required to show that there is no existing or satisfactory treatment, or that the new treatment offers a significant benefit over existing therapeutic interventions. We propose to compile all the available information in a single document, made available in a usable way to all Member States, so that member states would be able to coordinate their requests to the Marketing Authorisation Applicants: agreement on which minimum data set is required to understand the place of the product in the therapeutic strategy**.

Acknowledgements

Provenance Statement EURORDIS is a non-governmental patient-driven alliance of patient organisations and individuals active in the field of rare diseases, dedicated

[11] Improving access to orphan medicines for all affected EU citizens – Final Conclusions and Recommendations of the EU Pharmaceutical Forum – October 2008. http://ec.europa.eu/pharmaforum/docs/pricing_orphans_en.pdf.

to improving the quality of life of all people living with rare diseases in Europe. It was founded in 1997; it is supported by its members and by the French Muscular Dystrophy Association (AFM), the European Commission, and corporate foundations and the health industry.

EURORDIS represents more than 469 rare disease organisations in 41 different countries, covering approximately 4,000 distinct rare diseases.

The author has completed the Unified Competing Interest form at www.icmje.org/coi_disclosure.pdf (available on request from the corresponding author) and declare: no support from any organisation for the submitted work; Eurordis has received grants and honorariums from Amicus, Baxter, Amgen, CSL Behring, Sigma Tau Pharmaceuticals, Genzyme, Alexion, Biomarin, Boehringer Ingelheim, Chiesi Farmaceutici, Celgene, Fold Rx, Dompé farmaceutici, Glaxo Smith Kline, Gilead Sciences, Helsinn Health Care, IDM Pharma, Jerini, Laboratoire Français du Fractionnement et des Biotechnologies, Novartis,Orfagen, Orphan Europe, Pfizer, PharmaMar, PTC Therapeutics, Merck Serono International SA, Servier, Shire Pharmaceuticals, Talecris and Vifor Pharma; no other relationships or activities that could appear to have influenced the submitted work.

References

[1] Active involvement of patients in drug research, evaluation, and commercialization: European perspective, *Houyez F. J Ambul Care Manage* **27**(2) (Apr-Jun 2004), 139–145.

[2] Sébastien Dalgalarrondo "Quelle place pour les associations de malades dans le processus d'innovation médicamenteuse?", *Revue Française des Affaires sociales* 3/2007 (n° 3–4), pp. 171–191. URL: www.cairn.info/revue-francaise-des-affaires-sociales-2007-3-page-171.htm.

[3] QALYs: is the value of treatment proportional to the size of the health gain? Nord E, Enge AU, Gundersen V, *Health Econ* **19**(5) (May 2010), 596–607.

Pharmaceuticals Policy and Law 11 (2011) 177–181
DOI 10.3233/PPL-2011-0322
IOS Press

HTA's and access to rare diseases therapies: The view from the PID community

J. Prevot* and D. Watters
IPOPI, Downderry, Cornwall, UK

1. Introduction

When managing their healthcare budgets, governments and national agencies responsible for the provision of healthcare are faced with a number of challenges. Assessing the clinical effectiveness of a medicinal product or device should be the main factor on which decisions to reimburse or not reimburse a specific health technology should be made.

There are however many other factors that come into play. The rising costs of healthcare means that decision makers are increasingly implementing *cost containment measures* to reduce expenditure. Lobbying efforts by stakeholders, the political environment of a country and the willingness of healthcare management bodies to involve key stakeholders all are additional important considerations to take into account in the outcomes of an assessment procedure.

In the case of rare diseases therapies this intricate equation is further complicated by the fact that clinical efficacy data are harder to obtain due to the small patient populations who rely on these therapies. There are often no randomized clinical trials data available nor pharmacoeconomic data. However these therapies are often the only treatment available and can be life saving.

People living with primary immunodeficiencies (PID) represent such a patient population. Immunoglobulin replacement therapy is a life saving treatment derived from human plasma without which a large number of people living with PID would not be able to have a functional immune system and would be faced with recurrent life-impairing or life-threatening infections.

*Corresponding author: Johan Prévot, IPOPI, Firside, Main Road, Downderry, Cornwall PL11 3LE, UK. E-mail: johan@ipopi.org.

2. Primary immunodeficiencies

Primary immunodeficiencies refer to a group of approximately 200 rare disorders characterized by a deficient immune system. It is conservatively recognized that they are within the range of the European Union definition of a rare disease, < 1/2000 people.

PID are genetic or hereditary defects and can affect anyone regardless of age or sex. They vary in severity depending on whether one or several parts of the immune system are non functional (innate or adaptive). Failure of these systems can result in disease, and possible death, from infection with viruses as well as bacteria and fungi [1]. Primary immunodeficiencies are massively under-diagnosed, however once a diagnosis has been made and patients are treated with the appropriate therapy, people with PID can live a normal and productive life.

3. Health Technology Assessments

'Health Technology Assessments' is an increasingly used term which refers to the comparative evaluation of the effectiveness, the cost and other implications of a health technology, be it a medicinal product, medical device, diagnostic tool or other health systems. Whist the terminology (ie comparative effectiveness in the United States) and procedures referring to this method may vary from country to country; ultimately the goal is the same – reviewing the clinical and cost effectiveness of a health technology and granting reimbursement / reimbursement level or not. In simpler words, it is used to decide which patient gets what treatment or not.

One may assume that such assessment would be carried out when a new therapy is to be or has just been launched. However HTA assessments are also being increasingly used to review existing patient outcomes and the cost effectiveness of well established therapies. Haemophilia prophylaxis therapy currently under review by the Swedish HTA agency is an example.

4. HTA assessment and rare diseases therapies – the example of PID

HTA assessments of rare diseases therapies is made difficult by the fact that models that are applicable to more common medical conditions are not suited to small patient populations and seemingly 'costly' therapies. Randomized clinical trials and post marketing studies are rarely available for rare diseases, and alternative methods should be used by HTA agencies when reviewing their clinical effectiveness. Similarly classical pharmaco-economic models to measure the cost effectiveness of a given health technology are not often suitable to rare diseases therapies such as immunoglobulin replacement therapy for PID.

Whilst one could affirm that treatment for primary immunodeficiency is costly, this very cost should be put into the broader perspective and take into account other key implications and factors such as:

1. The impact of a therapy on the life expectancy and the quality of life of the patients
2. The impact in terms of societal and professional life (ie the cost to society related to inability to work and lead a productive life without treatment)
3. The impact of a restricted access to the appropriate therapy and the subsequent medical costs that would be incurred in the treatment of the symptoms rather than the cause of the symptoms.

Patients who have been diagnosed and are appropriately treated for their PID know better than anyone the societal benefits linked to optimal care. As Mrs Jose Drabwell once put it in an article: "Since I started on a routine of regular intravenous immunoglobulin infusions, I have had few problems, and I can honestly say that I have more energy, live life to the full, travel the world, work full time and I actually am healthier than many so called "healthy" people" [2].

Another telling quote from Ms Kathy Antilla similarly stated: "Years ago, a diagnosis of a primary immunodeficiency disease meant extremely compromised lives, not just for the patients, but for their families as well. With early diagnosis and access to appropriate therapies, many people diagnosed with this condition can live healthy, productive lives, like my son Isaac."

These factors should always be taken into account when making decisions that can potentially affect the quality of life and so should the macroeconomic impact which appropriate treatment and treatment levels will have, such as the increased contribution of patients to society, successful professional lives and reduction in hospital stays.

The cost of treatment once PID has been diagnosed should clearly be put into perspective with the financial burden of non- or misdiagnosis of PID and inappropriate treatment levels and their associated consequences (such as higher rates of infections, hospitalization, sick days and their resulting costs). It is well documented that "late diagnosis and delayed institution of immunoglobulin replacement therapy results in increased morbidity with a wide variety of organ-specific complications and increased mortality" [3].

Whilst this may seem obvious to any stakeholder involved in the primary immunodeficiency field, this message has to be voiced among healthcare budget decision makers.

This is why the involvement of stakeholders such as patient organisations in the HTA decision making process is absolutely necessary. IPOPI has engaged into a dialogue on HTAs and related assessment measures on the international level, such as through cooperation with other stakeholders on this edition of Pharmaceuticals Policy and Law, but it is crucial that such dialogue should be happening at the national level as well.

Whilst physicians should focus on collecting evidence based data, patient organisations can collect valuable experiential data looking at the broader meaning of living with a rare condition and the impact of therapy on many key aspects such quality of life, social, school and professional life as well as the impact of inappropriate treatment. In the field of primary immunodeficiencies such data has been collected so far in the United States of America by IPOPI's national member organisations, the Immune Deficiency Foundation (www.primaryimmune.org) and the Jeffrey Modell Foundation (http://www.info4pi.org).

It has for example been demonstrated in a study conducted by IDF in the US that "once [PID] patients begin receiving IVIG on a regular basis their health status improves markedly, their activity limitations drop significantly and their quality of life improves dramatically" [4]. In another US study led by the Jeffrey Modell Foundation, it was demonstrated that "each undiagnosed patient with an underlying Primary Immunodeficiency disease costs the healthcare system an average of $102,736 annually. Each diagnosed patient with a recognized Primary Immunodeficiency disease costs the healthcare system an average of $22,696 annually. (....) The economic impact of undiagnosed Primary Immunodeficiency patients to the healthcare system in the United States totals over $40 billion annually" [5].

These survey outcomes attest to the undeniable value of early diagnosis and optimal treatment of patients living with a primary immunodeficiency.

5. Conclusions

As HTA assessments and similar mechanisms such as comparative effectiveness are increasingly being used to guide healthcare budgetary decisions, it is imperative for the PID stakeholders community to continue to collect data to ensure that should these assessments be applied to replacement therapy for PID patients, the arguments developed in this article and so well known by physicians, patient groups, nursing groups and industry can be appropriately be incorporated into the HTA process. A close collaboration between key stakeholders to ensure that experiential data and evidence-based data demonstrating the societal and broader economic value of early diagnosis of PID and appropriate treatment is needed more than ever before. Whilst further studies on the value of immunoglobulin therapy in the treatment of PID are necessary, additional studies are likely to be needed for other treatment options such as bone marrow transplantation and future use of gene therapy and monoclonal antibody therapies for some specific immunodeficiencies. As cost containment measures on healthcare budgets are likely to keep increasing, IPOPI is committed to work on this topic in the future to ensure that the broader societal and macro economic impact of PID treatment is taken into account into the health technology assessments process.

International and EU level initiatives that seek to involve key stakeholders such as patient organisations into the HTA process are fortunately taking place through bodies such as HTAi and EUnetHTA. The latter defines HTA as 'a multidisciplinary process that summarises information about the medical, social, economic and ethical issues related to the use of a health technology in a systematic, transparent, un-biased, robust manner. Its aim is to inform the formulation of safe, effective, health policies that are patient focused and seek to achieve best value. Despite its policy goals, HTA must always be firmly rooted in research and the scientific method" [6]. Whilst this definition is an excellent one, it seems that it is somewhat much more of a utopia or an objective to reach in the years to come than a description of how HTAs are currently being carried out. There is an increasing recognition by such bodies and stakeholder think tanks such as EPPOSI that societal impact must be incorporated into the HTA process. In conclusion, it would be wrong to dissociate the costs of a given treatment from the benefits that a healthier population will bring in return to society. As the saying goes, "Health is wealth".

References

[1] H. Chapel and P.D. Arkwright, *What are Immunodeficiencies?* Pharmaceuticals Policy and Law, Volume 10, 2008.
[2] J. Drabwell, *Living life to the fullest*, Pharmaceuticals Policy and Law, Volume 10, 2008.
[3] P. Wood, *The value of early diagnosis and treatment of patients with Primary Antibody Deficiencies*, Pharmaceuticals Policy and Law, Volume 10, 2008.
[4] M.L. Boyle and C. Scalchunes, *Impact of IVIG treatment among Patients with Primary Immunodeficiency Diseases*, Pharmaceuticals Policy and Law, Volume 10, 2008.
[5] J. Modell, *Primary Immunodeficiencies The Importance of Earliest Possible Diagnosis*, Pharmaceuticals Policy and Law, Volume 10, 2008.
[6] EUnetHTA, http://www.eunethta.eu/Public/About_EUnetHTA/HTA/.

Pharmaceuticals Policy and Law 13 (2011) 183–191
DOI 10.3233/PPL-2011-0323
IOS Press

Comparative effectiveness research in the United States and primary immunodeficiency diseases

Emily Hovermale*, Christopher Scalchunes and Marcia Boyle
Immune Deficiency Foundation, Towson, MD, USA

The United States enacted legislation in 2010 that will promote the use of comparative effectiveness research in the making of healthcare decisions. Of concern with this relatively new mandate is the possibility of using comparative effectiveness research as a means only to mitigate costs rather than to focus on quality of care. This is of particular concern for patients with rare and chronic conditions, such as primary immunodeficiency diseases. The Immune Deficiency Foundation (IDF) uses their survey research to advocate for the needs of patients with primary immunodeficiency diseases to ensure that their unique medical concerns are not overlooked but instead, integrated within an overall healthcare emphasis on personalized medicine and differences in patient treatment response. IDF research shows the efficacy of treatment with immunoglobulin replacement therapy (IG therapy) for many patients with primary immunodeficiency diseases, that IG therapy is underused in the primary immunodeficient community, and that IG therapies are unique and not interchangeable.

Keywords: Comparative effectiveness research, primary immunodeficiency diseases, Immune Deficiency Foundation, IDF, immunoglobulin therapy, IG therapy

1. Background

Primary immunodeficiency diseases (PIDD) represent a class of disorders in which there is an intrinsic defect in the immune system (rather than immune disorders that are secondary to infection, chemotherapy, or some other external agent). In some cases, the body fails to produce any or enough antibodies to fight infection. In other cases, the cellular, phagocytic or complement defenses against infection fail to work properly. There are more than 150 different primary immunodeficiency diseases currently recognized by the World Health Organization [1]. In 2005, the Immune Deficiency Foundation (IDF) commissioned a survey to help establish an estimated prevalence of PIDD in the United States. A national probability sample of 10,000 households was sampled by random digit dialing and screened by telephone to identify how many of the nearly 27,000 household members had been diagnosed with a PIDD. This study yielded an estimated population prevalence of diagnosed primary immunodeficiency diseases at 1 in 1,200 persons in the United States. When applied to the U.S. population of 311,656,000 persons, this suggests approximately

*Corresponding author: Emily Hovermale, Immune Deficiency Foundation, 40 W. Chesapeake Ave, Ste 308, Towson, MD, USA. Tel.: +1 410 321 6647; E-mail: ehovermale@primaryimmune.org.

250,000 persons have a diagnosed primary immunodeficiency disease in the United States [2]. Many individuals with a PIDD receive treatment through infusions of immunoglobulin therapy, an effective replacement therapy for the antibody deficiency forms of the disease. Today, immunoglobulin replacement therapy is available in intravenous (IVIG) and subcutaneous (SCIG) modes of administration.

2. Comparative effectiveness research in the United States and the PIDD population

The Patient Protection and Affordable Care Act (PPACA), enacted in March 2010, established the Patient-Centered Outcomes Research Institute (the Institute), a private, non-profit entity that will establish research priorities, fund comparative clinical effectiveness research, train researchers in comparative effectiveness research methods, communicate results to the public, and in general provide for the conduct of comparative effectiveness research. The legislation requires that the Institute ensure that diversity in populations is accounted for in research designs. The law also prohibits any findings of comparative effectiveness research to be construed as practice guidelines or coverage decisions and contains safeguards for patients against discriminatory coverage decisions [3]. The Institute is operational and currently conducting a schedule of public meetings.

IDF is the national patient organization dedicated to improving the diagnosis, treatment and quality of life of persons with PIDD in the United States. During federal legislation negotiations, IDF actively advocated for the legislation to appropriately leave key health care decisions up to patients and their physicians, and not to their insurers, by ensuring that the Institute's research focused on quality care rather than on cost. Due to the complex health care needs of persons with PIDD, a "one size fits all" approach is never appropriate for this patient population. Rather, health care should focus on the patient's needs and specific concerns and medical issues, which may be affected by that individual's co-morbidities, sex, race, or other key factors.

As patient advocates, IDF, in collaboration the American Plasma Users Coalition (A-PLUS), worked with the United States Congress to ensure that the law provides patients with key information for making health care decisions, including provisions to ensure that funding is available to disseminate key research findings. A-PLUS is a coalition of rare disease patient organizations whose patients rely on plasma-derived products to live relatively healthy and productive lives with chronic conditions. IDF and A-PLUS appreciate that the law assures that the key research elements – from the beginning of the design phases – are publicly available for review. It is hoped that this open, transparent process will provide a research avenue on key issues specific to patients, especially those with rare diseases, before proceeding with comparative effectiveness research.

Importantly, IDF and the rare disease community worked with Congress to ensure that the Institute is required to establish and consult with an Expert Advisory Panel for

Rare Diseases. The Panel will assist in the design of research studies and determine the relative value and feasibility of conducting particular research studies.

An ongoing concern in the United States related to comparative effectiveness research is its potential use to limit care. This is of particular concern to patients with rare, chronic diseases who have especially complex medical needs and resulting high medical costs. To address this concern, the law states that the Institute may not mandate coverage, reimbursement, or other policies for any public or private payer. Also, the U.S. Secretary of Health and Human Services is prohibited from using the Institute's research in determining coverage, or creating reimbursement or incentive programs for a treatment in ways that (1) treat extending the life of an elderly, disabled, or terminally ill patient of lower value than extending the life of others or (2) preclude or discourage an individual from choosing a health care treatment based on how the individual values the tradeoff between extending the length of their life and the risk of disability [3].

In the United States Congress, legislation continues to be introduced to protect against rationing of care linked to the Institute. For example, Senator Kyl (R-AZ) introduced S. 660, the "Preserving Access to Targeted, Individualized, and Effective New Treatments and Services (PATIENTS) Act of 2011," with the stated purpose to "protect all patients by prohibiting the use of data obtained from comparative effectiveness research to deny or delay coverage of items or services under Federal health care programs and to ensure that comparative effectiveness research accounts for advancements in personalized medicine and differences in patient treatment response" [4].

3. Medical characteristics of patients with PIDD

IDF is concerned with the lack of research conducted on behalf of rare and chronic disease populations, particularly for patients with primary immunodeficiency diseases. The major health surveys conducted by the government in the United States–the National Health Interview Survey and the National Health and Nutrition Examination Survey–do not collect information on primary immunodeficiency diseases. No comprehensive population survey has ever been undertaken by the federal government to estimate the prevalence or the population characteristics of these diseases in the United States. Thus, research conducted by IDF has focused on filling the data gap with regard to individuals with PIDD so that information on the characteristics and what constitutes quality of care for this population is available. IDF has conducted a series of surveys including three *National Patient Surveys* and three *Treatment Experiences and Preferences of Patients with Primary Immune Deficiency Diseases Surveys* in the effort to create a comprehensive portrait of the primary immunodeficienct patient, their medical condition and their treatment.

The majority of patients with a diagnosis of a PIDD who respond to IDF surveys have an antibody deficiency for which immunoglobulin therapy is the standard of care.

The IDF treatment surveys are based on a large sample of persons known to IDF who use immunoglobulin replacement therapy in the treatment of their PIDD. All three of these are nationally distributed surveys, each with more than 1,000 completions. These cases provide a relatively large national sample of persons with PIDD who have been treated with IG therapy. Although these surveys are not probability samples from which we can make population estimates within known limits of sampling error, they provide the most representative samples currently available of patients with a rare disease from which we can examine treatment experiences.

The Second and Third National Treatment Experiences and Preferences of Patients with Primary Immunodeficiency Diseases Surveys provide data on the treatment of patients with PIDD including the patients' needs, specific concerns and medical issues. The data from these surveys showed that the average time to diagnosis from symptom onset for this population is between 9–13.4 years [5,6]. This extended period of time without diagnosis, and thus without effective treatment, resulted in more complex treatment needs as additional medical issues increased for the PIDD patient population. Analysis from the *2007 IDF National Patient Survey* indicates that there is a positive correlation between time to diagnosis as primary immune deficient and the number of permanent functional impairments (Pearson's $r(1127) = 0.301, p < 0.001$).

As a result of late diagnosis, and repeated and severe infections prior to diagnosis, over one half of patients with PIDD reported at least some permanent impairment before their diagnosis as immune deficient. This complicates a number of systems and functions within the body. Nearly two out of five patients with PIDD reported permanent impairment of lung function (37%) prior to diagnosis. Additionally, 17% had permanent impairment to digestive function, 13% hearing loss or impairment, 8% neurological impairment, 7% loss of mobility, and 5% had either vision loss or impairment. Another 11% had some other permanent impairment or loss prior to diagnosis as immune deficient [6].

4. Efficacy of immunoglobulin replacement therapy in treating PIDD

The data cited in Boyle and Scalchunes' article in *Pharmaceuticals Policy and Law* based on past IDF surveys not only illustrates the specific medical issues of this population, but also highlights the use of IG therapy as an effective treatment for the majority of patients with PIDD, which greatly improves the health and quality of life of these patients. To best measure the efficacy of IG therapy among patients, a series of questions were asked to gauge the health of the patient in the twelve months prior to diagnosis and in the twelve months most recent to the survey. The comparison in health status provides the most compelling evidence of the efficacy of IG therapy to control PIDD and demonstrates the improvement in the health and well-being of the patient since treatment had begun. Prior to diagnosis, less than one-in-five patients with PIDD who used IG therapy described their health status as excellent (4%), very good (4%) or good (11%). However, in the twelve months most recent to the survey, the same patients with PIDD described their health status in a much more positive way. Three-quarters of patients with PIDD using IVIG therapy described their health in the 12 months most recent to the survey as excellent (16%) very good (28%) or good (29%) [7].

One reason that most patients with PIDD described their health as good or better in the 12 months prior to the survey, compared to the 12 months prior to treatment, was a lower incidence of chronic and acute infections associated with PIDD. These patients reported a decrease in many chronic conditions, including a decrease in pneumonia (51% prior to diagnosis, 13% recent), bronchitis (56% prior, 34% recent), and ear infections (47% prior, 27% recent) [7]. IG therapy for patients with PIDD translates into improved quality of life and better health outcomes for these individuals. Fifty-seven percent of patients with PIDD reported being hospitalized during the year prior to their diagnosis. In contrast, only 25% reported a hospitalization in the year most recent to the survey. When diagnosed patients do go to the hospital, they spend less time there. Patients reported an average number of nights in the hospital of 9.2 in the year prior to diagnosis versus only 4.3 nights in the year most recent to the survey [7].

5. Underuse of immunoglobulin replacement therapy in treating PIDD

Despite the overwhelming evidence of the efficacy of IG therapy for patients with PIDD, IDF survey data has also shown that underuse of IG therapy for these conditions persists. In the two most recent IDF national surveys of patients known to the Foundation, *Primary Immune Deficiency Diseases In America*, IDF found that two-thirds of patients with a PIDD were using intravenous immunoglobulin for their condition [8,9]. Boyle and Buckley's article in the *Journal of Clinical Immunology* based on research conducted by IDF indicated that there might be a serious problem with underuse of IG therapy in the treatment of PIDD. Although 57% of the patients in this survey had a PIDD diagnosis for which IG therapy is the standard of care, only 22% of these patients from the national household telephone survey were currently being treated with immunoglobulin for their disease [2]. This estimate of 22% is based on a very small sample size. In order to examine the rates of immunoglobulin therapy in a large, national sample of patients diagnosed with PIDD, IDF conducted an Internet survey in 2010 using a national online general population panel that sent more than 850,000 invitations to participate. Based on this national survey, the data shows that less than half of patients with PIDD who have a diagnosis for which IG therapy is recommended (46%) are currently being treated with any form of immunoglobulin therapy [10].

This suggests that a substantial segment of patients with PIDD are being under-treated for their condition compared to clinical guidelines and thus put at increased risk for more health concerns. As expected, the patients with PIDD in this national sample also reported generally lower health status than those found in previous IDF patient surveys based on patients in the IDF database where the percentage of those using IG therapy was higher. These poorer health outcomes of patients in the Internet survey, compared to surveys of patients in the IDF's databases, may be related to the lower rates of IG therapy for patients with PIDD in the general population [9,10].

Among the patients with PIDD in the *National Internet Treatment Survey of Primary Immunodeficiency Diseases in the United States*, who had previously been treated with IG therapy but were no longer receiving these treatments, the most common reasons for cessation of treatment were that the product was too expensive (43%), lack of insurance (29%), or difficulty in obtaining the product (29%) [10]. In the case of access to appropriate treatment for patients with PIDD, this data shows that in some cases cost supersedes quality of care. In order to better understand how primary care physicians are diagnosing, managing and treating patients with primary immunodeficiencies, IDF conducted national mail surveys of pediatricians and family practitioners. Results from these surveys indicate a lack of understanding by many of these physicians as to the efficacy and safety of IG therapy as treatment for patients with antibody deficiencies (unpublished results, manuscript in preparation). It is likely that in many instances, this leads to less than optimal health outcomes for patients with PIDD under the care of these physicians.

6. Patients tolerate immunoglobulin replacement therapies differently

IDF data also confirms the research done by others in the field showing the importance of individualized medicine and differences in treatment responses for patients with PIDD who are treated with immunoglobulin replacement therapy. While all immunoglobulin therapies available on the US market are approved by the Food and Drug Administration (FDA) and clinically effective in treating patients with PIDD for which IG therapy is indicated, there are currently no generic or equivalent versions of IG. Rather, a number of factors impact how an individual patient will tolerate and respond to a particular brand of immunoglobulin, including the patient's medical history and the product's characteristics such as the volume delivered, sugar content, IgA content, pH, route of administration and osmolality. The FDA requires that an individual clinical trial protocol is completed for each immunoglobulin product to receive licensure, even if it is from the same manufacturer, effectively recognizing that each product is unique and not interchangeable [11]. Manufacturing differences can, and do, affect individuals' tolerability, risk of adverse events, infusion rate, and potential efficacy [12].

The Third National Treatment Experiences and Preferences of Patients with Primary Immunodeficiency Diseases Survey found that 41% of the patients surveyed reported tolerating some IG therapy products better than others. Of those who reported having a serious side effect or reaction to their IG therapy, 28% reported having a serious side-effect or reaction when they tried a new IG product for the first time and 13% had a serious side effect or reaction when they switched products [6].

Adverse reactions can range in severity from redness at the infusion site and severe headaches to anaphylaxis, kidney failure – and even death. As a result of the data and the clinical experience of some of the nation's leading immunologists, the leading body of specialists in immunology, the American Academy of Allergy, Asthma and Immunology (AAAAI), included a principle in the *AAAAI Eight Guiding Principles for Appropriate Use of IVIG for Primary Immunodeficiency Diseases* stating that IVIG is not a generic drug and IVIG products are not interchangeable [13].

The data reported by IDF showing the difference in treatment responses to IG therapy is supported by Feldmeyer et al who report that 35% of patients in their study experience mild or moderate adverse reactions during or within 48 hours of the administration of a standard IVIG preparation which did not recur after switching to an alternative preparation [14]. Similarly, Dashti-Khavidaki et al found in their study of patients with primary immunodeficiency disease over a 13 year period that "34 out of 216 [roughly 15%] of adverse reactions were caused by a change in the IVIG product" [15]. Amertunga, Sinclair, & Kolbe also report in their study that a change in IVIG formulation of a specific product resulted in adverse reactions by seven of the 49 (roughly 14.2%) patients involved in the study [16]. This body of research speaks to the need for personalized medicine with regard to the complex health care needs of patients with PIDD.

While the inclination of some insurers may be to treat IG therapies as generic and interchangeable with the goal of instituting cost cutting formularies, this is not a viable option for patient safety. Not only may the health of patients be negatively impacted if these individuals are switched with no medical justification, but instituting a policy that treats IG therapies as generic is also an unwise cost option. There is no way to predict which patients will have an adverse event or how serious the adverse event will be when switching a patient to a product that they have never before used. There is no question that instituting such a policy will result in increased cost in some patients due to additional medical treatment for patients who experience adverse events.

7. Conclusion

With the continued emphasis on reducing healthcare costs in the United States, there is concern that comparative effectiveness research could be used as justification for instituting health care protocols that focus on cost containment rather than quality of care. This is of particular concern for patients who, like those with primary immunodeficiency diseases, have rare and chronic conditions. IDF research illustrates the efficacy of treatment with immunoglobulin replacement therapy (IG therapy) for many patients with primary immunodeficiency diseases. The research also shows that IG therapy is underused in the primary immunodeficient community as a result of cost and lack of insurance coverage, as well as physician and patient lack of awareness. It is important to note that immunoglobulin replacement therapy products are unique and tolerated differently by different patients. Attempts to treat these therapies as generic, with the hope of containing costs, will be detrimental to patient safety.

IDF will continue to monitor the activities of the Patient-Centered Outcomes Research Institute as well as efforts, such as formularies, by insurance companies to contain costs. At the same time, IDF will use its research to advocate for the needs of patients with primary immunodeficiency diseases and ensure that their unique medical concerns are integrated within an overall health care emphasis on personalized medicine.

References

[1] L. Notarangelo, J. Casanova, M. Conley, M. Chapel, A. Fischer, J. Puck et al., Primary immunodeficiency diseases: an update from the International Union of Immunological Societies Primary Immunodeficiency Diseases Classification Committee Meeting in Budapest, 2005, *J Allergy Clin Immunol* **117** (2006), 883–896.

[2] J.M. Boyle and R.H. Buckley, Population Prevalence of Diagnosed Primary Immunodeficiency Diseases in the United States, *J Clin Immunol* **27** (2007), 497–502.

[3] Patient Protection and Affordable Care Act, Pub. L. 111-148 (2010).

[4] Preserving Access to Targeted, Individualized, and Effective New Treatments and Services (PATIENTS) Act of 2011, S. 660, 112th Cong. (2011).

[5] IDF (Immune Deficiency Foundation). Treatment Experiences and Preferences of Patients with Primary Immune Deficiency Diseases: 2002 – The Second National Treatment Survey of Patients. Prepared by Schulman, Ronca & Bucuvalas, Inc. June 2003.

[6] IDF (Immune Deficiency Foundation). Treatment Experiences and Preferences among Patients with Primary Immunodeficiency Diseases: 2008 – The Third National Treatment Survey of Patients. Prepared by Abt SRBI, Inc. May 2009.

[7] M. Boyle and C. Scalchunes, Impact of Intravenous Immunoglobulin (IVIG) treatment among patients with Primary Immunodeficiency diseases, *Pharmaceuticals Policy and Law* **10** (2008), 133–146.

[8] IDF (Immune Deficiency Foundation). Primary Immune Deficiency Diseases in America: 2002 – The Second National Survey of Patients. Prepared by Schulman, Ronca & Bucuvalas, Inc. April 2003.

[9] IDF (Immune Deficiency Foundation). Primary Immunodeficiency Diseases in America: 2007 – The Third National Survey of Patients. Prepared by Abt SRBI, Inc. May 2009.

[10] IDF (Immune Deficiency Foundation). National Internet Treatment Survey of Primary Immunodeficiency Diseases in the United States. Prepared by Abt SRBI, Inc. July 2010.

[11] U.S. Food and Drug Administration: *Immunoglobulin intravenous (IGIV) indications, 2007.* Retrieved June 30, 2011 from http://www.fda.gov/BiologicsBloodVaccines/BloodBloodProducts/ApprovedProducts/LicensedProductsBLAs/FractionatedPlasmaProducts/ucm133691.htm.

[12] J. Siegel, The Product: All intravenous immunoglobulins are not equivalent, *Pharmacotherapy* **25**(11 pt2) (2005), 785–845.

[13] American Academy of Allergy Asthma and Immunology eight guiding principles for the safe, effective and appropriate use of IVIG for PI. Retrieved June 30, 2011from http://www.aaaai.org/members/resources/initiatives/ivig_toolkit/ivig_coverage.pdf.

[14] L. Feldmeyer, C. Benden, S. Haile, A. Boehler, R. Speich, L. French and G. Hofmauer, Not all intravenous immunoglobulin preparations are equally well tolerated, *Acta Derm Venereol* **90** (2010), 494–497.

[15] S. Dashti-Khavidak, A. Aghamohammadi, F. Farshadi, M. Movahedi, N. Parvaneh, N. Pouladi, K. Moazzami, T. Cheraghi, S. Mahdaviani, S. Saghafi, G. Heydari, A. Abdollahzade and N. Rezaei,

Adverse reactions of prophylactic intravenous immunoglobulin; A 13 year experience with 3004 infusions in Iranian patients with primary immunodeficiency diseases, *J investing Allergol Clin Immunol* **19**(2) (2009), 139–145.
[16] R. Amertunga, J. Sinclair and J. Kolbe, Increased risk of adverse events when changing intravenous immunoglobulin preparations, *Clin Exp Immunol* **136** (2004), 111–113

Pharmaceuticals Policy and Law 13 (2011) 193–201
DOI 10.3233/PPL-2011-0324
IOS Press

Patient engagement in health technology assessment (HTA)

Report on the 2nd Epposi Workshop, and next steps*

Jacqueline Bowman-Busato
Epposi, 21 rue Marie-Thérèse, B-1000 Brussels, Belgium
Tel.: +32 (0)2 503 1307; E-mail: jacqueline.bowman@epposi.org

Epposi is an independent, not-for-profit, partnership-led and multi-stakeholder think tank based in Brussels, Belgium, committed to supporting the realisation of the EU-2020 strategic vision through the health and wellbeing of its citizens.

Our Goal is to work at the "cutting edge" of European health policy-making providing members and the wider public with high-quality independent research, capacity-building, knowledge exchange and dissemination with the aim of bridging the gap between innovation and improved public health outcomes. Membership is equally weighted between academic sciences, industry and patient organisations.

1. Introduction

Health technology assessment (HTA) – a multidisciplinary field of policy analysis that studies the medical, social, ethical, and economic implications of the development, diffusion and use of health technology – is increasingly playing a central role in how national healthcare priorities are set and service provision is delivered in most EU member states.

It should benefit both patients and healthcare payers by allowing faster, evidence-based access to innovative technologies that are clinically sound and cost-effective, while helping to eliminate treatments and practices that are shown to deliver limited health benefits or financial value. However, the role of the patient in the HTA process is often ill defined, with widely varying criteria on which HTA decisions are based being applied in EU Member States, which can lead to inequality of access to treatment.

1.1. The role of patients in HTA

In order to increase the understanding of the contribution that patients and patient organisations can make to HTA, Epposi, a Brussels-based multi-stakeholder health

*This article is an abridged version of the full report of the workshop held on 17 November 2010 in Brussels, Belgium.

innovation think tank, organised a two-stage workshop. The first part took place in Brussels on 29 June 2010 and brought together an invited group of experts representing all stakeholder groups to explore the context in which HTA is currently undertaken and how "patient engagement" can play a greater role within it.

The participants concluded that patients' participation in HTA is invaluable as they provide unique perspectives and real-life experience which can:

- inform the translation of evidence of efficacy (such as clinical trial results) towards the concept of effectiveness (actual experience)
- inform economic models based on delineating disease pathways, treatment preferences and the burden of disease
- provide crucial insights into living with the disease and unmet needs that inform value judgments in the deliberative process.

To encourage the effective participation of patients in HTA, it was agreed that a follow-up workshop would be needed to draw up the key elements of consensus guidelines which could be developed into concrete recommendations and promoted to national agencies, the European Commission/EUnetHTA and international organisations such as HTAi.

The follow-up workshop was held on 17 November 2010 in Brussels and attracted nearly 80 attendees representing patients' associations, payers, EU and national policy-makers in public health, HTA and ICT, healthcare professions, pharmaceutical and medical diagnostics industries, academic sciences and research.

Participants focused their discussions on four main questions from which they set out to elicit recommendations to improve patient engagement in HTA:

1. How should we engage with patients to ensure that HTA is truly patient-centred and when and how should patients engage in the HTA process?
2. What questions can patients ask of the "hard" evidence to be sure that it reflects their concerns?
3. How can patient organisations collect evidence that will be useful for HTAs?
4. What can HTA agencies do to improve engagement with patients?

The European Commission and EU Member States have attempted to clarify what can be better achieved on HTA at EU level by setting up EUnetHTA, a Joint Action network of 34 government-appointed organisations from the EU Member States, accession countries and EEA (European Economic Area), which runs from January 2010 to 2012.

Finn Børlum Kristensen, Chairman of the Executive Committee of the EUnetHTA and a speaker at Epposi's November workshop, endorsed the need for HTA agencies to do more to support patient engagement: "It's my view that all agencies should have policies for patient involvement. There is a clear need for more transparency on the work of agencies and clear indications on where patient engagement should take place."

2. Setting the framework to allow multi-stakeholder perspectives

The opening panel debate, chaired by Hilda Bastian, Head of the Health Information Department of IQWIG (Germany's HTA agency – Institute for Quality and Efficiency in Health Care), outlined the key challenges to ensuring greater patient participation in HTA from the perspectives of patients – represented by Yann Le Cam, CEO of EURORDIS (Rare Diseases Europe) – science and academia, by Prof Helle Ploug-Hansen of the Institute of Public Health Research Unit: Health, Environment & Society, University of Southern Denmark – and industry, by Maria Fagerquist of EFPIA (European Federation of Pharmaceutical Industries and Associations).

2.1. Science

Prof Ploug-Hansen emphasised the importance of using multiple research methodologies to ensure that patients' wider perspectives are taken into account – qualitative studies, quantitative studies, syntheses of qualitative studies and literature reviews (even unpublished studies where relevant) – to deepen knowledge and produce more rounded and robust evidence. She also made the point that in HTA contexts, the term 'patient' can also refer to 'citizen', 'customer', 'user' and 'individual'.

She advocated a more anthropological approach to the collection of evidence to include the wider psycho-social aspects of patients' daily lives which impact on how they deal with their disease or condition and which help strengthen best practice. Depending on the context, the answers elicited can be very different: for example, whether the patient is in hospital or at home, the kinds of care and support networks in place and so on. However, she emphasised that it is the researchers who must interpret the data but the processes must be transparent so that both the patients and researchers' perspectives and roles are clear.

2.2. Industry

Drawing on her former experience at the Swedish Pricing and Reimbursement Authority (TLV) – an agency that applies HTA in its decision-making – Maria Fagerquist asserted the right of patients to be involved in HTA as not only democratic but irrefutable, commenting that "you cannot possibly exclude arguably the most central stakeholder from the process." Not only are they the only ones to know the full implications of a disease and its treatment but a greater sense of engagement leads to greater commitment to treatment. Effectiveness – a key determinant of HTA - is based on the actual use of medicines so patients' preferences should therefore be an integral part of assessments, she argued.

She cited three examples of good practice:

- **Sweden** – patient representatives participate as members of expert groups of the Swedish Council on Health Technology Assessment (SBU) on equal terms as other clinical and pharmaceutical experts. The patient representative provides a patient perspective on ethical considerations, as well as interpreting and assessing the reasonableness of study outcomes.

- **Scotland** – Scottish Medicines Consortium (SMC) has an online web-based patient submission system which is prepared by Patient Interest Groups which collect comments from patients and carers. A user-friendly patient submission template has been created to make it easier for patients to share their experiences and give their perspective on a range of issues, including how medicine meets patients' needs; the advantages/disadvantages over other available medicines; and how the medicine impacts on patients/carers' lives
- **Australia** – consumer impact statements are sought to find out what impact a disease has on the daily life of patients and there is a consumer representative on the PBAC (Pharmaceutical Benefits Advisory Committee) who has advance notice of and input in the agenda.

However, overall, she concluded, progress was patchy with too few examples of successful patient involvement at the level of "setting the process" and stressed that patients need training and support to be fully involved.

2.3. Patients

Yann Le Cam argued that only patients can offer a truly all-encompassing perspective on all aspects essential to good HTA decisions. Patients are the only people with direct, real-life experience of living with a particular disease and able to closely monitor the true effects of drug therapies and dosages. They also know the daily practicalities of navigating health systems and administrations, medical practices and care networks, so it is essential that they are involved. He also noted that patients have already gained a lot of experience in participating in other European health regulatory areas, such as in EMA (European Medicines Agency) and on pharmaco-vigilance issues, which is leading to better outcomes.

This unique perspective offered crucial added value across HTA processes, he believed, from helping to improve the design of trials, recruitment and end points to the interpretation of data.

As further evidence, he offered two additional benefits of patient involvement:

1. self-reported outcomes on risks, benefits and effectiveness, which are very important before and after marketing authorisation, and working with regulatory agencies
2. studies of patients' treatment preferences which can provide a bridge between EMA and HTA at national levels.

Much more needs to be done to experiment with and expand on these methodologies, he urged. But there is much that is happening: in the field of orphan drugs, he noted that there is now 10 years of evidence since the EU directive came into effect to endorse reimbursement decisions at national level; DG Enterprise & Industry has launched a two-year process looking at conditional pricing; and EURORDIS is now offering a training programme on HTA to create critical mass and skills so patients can really participate nationally and in EUnetHTA.

3. Addressing the challenges: 4 key questions

To address the four key questions outlined in the objectives, the participants divided into four breakout groups, maintaining a strict stakeholder balance in each.

3.1. How should we engage with patients to ensure that HTA is truly patient-centred and when and how should patients engage in the HTA process?

The session was chaired by Dr Karen Facey of Health Technology Assessment International (HTAi) and Yann Le Cam of EURORDIS. The discussions centred on the need for the clear recognition of the value of patients' perspectives and to obtain a clear commitment to include patient involvement at all levels: governance, committees, technology and medicine where HTA processes are involved. It was noted that EUnetHTA has a stakeholder involvement policy (not just for patients) and that it would be helpful if each HTA Agency had a patient involvement policy that clearly outlined how patients' perspectives were sought and how patients and patient organisations could get involved in the HTA process.

How should this be done? Patients should be involved in scoping the HTA and submission of evidence (using social media and networking, self-reported outcomes, patient preferences and patient organisation databases). HTA agencies should support patient organisations to understand the type of information that is valuable.

Table 1
How and when should patients be engaged in the HTA process?

Summary of Main Findings
1. All HTA agencies in Europe should have a policy that presents how they involve patients and patient evidence in their HTA process. Ideally this should be based on a minimum set of actions to engage patients in their work and ensure that their views are taken account of in decision-making.
2. To promote education on HTA on how to get involved as a patient representative to add value to the system.
3. Good starting points: The International Network of Agencies for HTA has already performed a survey of consumer involvement in HTA agencies and is in the process of doing another. The European Patients' Forum is undertaking a survey of agencies and patient organisations in Europe to determine involvement. EFPIA is also conducting research into patient involvement in HTA processes and EUnetHTA is creating a core model for HTA that includes consideration of patient issues. Epposi might want to consider activities that promote collaboration among these groups.

Proper training is also important but it was agreed that the key point is that this must be organised by patient groups and not by HTA agencies but to have staff from HTA agencies involved. HTAi has developed a glossary for patients and promotes a Patient's Guide to HTA. HTA agencies also need to organise regular sessions to introduce themselves to patient organisations in their countries, explain what they do and how their processes work.

3.2. What questions can patients ask of the "hard" evidence to be sure that it reflects their concerns?

The session was chaired by Prof Helle Ploug-Hansen of the University of Southern Denmark and Maarten de Wit of the Dutch League of Arthritis Patients' Associations.

The group discussed the too narrow focus of most HTA agencies on 'hard' evidence criteria (mainly based on clinical trials) which exclude patients' real-life daily experiences and other important factors such as family life and care networks, the work environment and social life.

In the participants' view, HTA agencies needed stronger and clearer structures to allow the consideration of evidence based on both qualitative and quantitative research methods and to provide patients' representatives with adequate support and training to enable them to participate on an equal footing with other relevant stakeholders. This would also help to mitigate any potential safety issues inherent in 'softer' evidence, as well as allow national and regional differences to be taken into account.

Table 2
What questions can patients ask of the "hard" evidence?

Summary of Main Findings
1. Good guidance is lacking not just for patients but also for researchers.
2. HTA agencies should take full account of societal and cultural aspects.
3. HTA agencies should provide training for patients and researchers on how to collaborate in an HTA process. Competences to achieve this do not come automatically.
4. Strong wish from patients' organisations for Epposi to create a European Charter for patients to have fair access.

3.3. How can patient organisations collect evidence that will be useful for HTAs?

The session was chaired by Liuska Sanna of the European Patients' Forum and Andrea Rappagliosi of GSK. The discussions uncovered a wide range of questions and challenges, including the difficulties for patient organisations to gather the evidence and knowing what HTA agencies are actually looking for; the difficulties for patient organisations to format the information for the purposes of the HTA so it can be standardised and how 'soft', more anecdotal, data on patients' daily experience can be incorporated; the independence of evidence provided – who pays to help patient

Table 3
How can patient organisations collect evidence that will be useful for HTAs?

Summary of Main Findings
1. Foster the early engagement of patient organisations in clinical trials to integrate quality of life, social and ethical information into the evidence-collection for HTA agencies. 2. Involve patient organisations in gathering data post-marketing authorisation to inform long-term relative effectiveness assessments.

organisations collect evidence and transparency issues; knowing which methodologies/approaches patient organisations can use to collect and present evidence; and getting HTA agencies to take into account patients' preferences and their own value judgments on treatment methods.

3.4. What can HTA agencies do to improve engagement with patients?

The session was chaired by Alastair Kent of Genetic Alliance UK and Lizzie Amis of NICE (National Institute for Health and Clinical Excellence, England). The group noted that before HTA agencies can improve engagement with patients they must secure political engagement to ensure trust and effectiveness, as well as high-level policy agreement on the engagement of patients at all levels.

Other key challenges highlighted during the discussions included the need for clear, two-way channels of communication and information between agencies and patients, where patients are consulted (early), treated as experts and given equal status as other decision-makers in HTA processes. Transparency was also key so that all stakeholders – policy-makers, patients, academics and industry – understood the process and knew what was expected of them, when and why.

The participants also raised the importance of quality of life issues and the need for cost issues to be broadened to look at the costs to society as a whole, not just to the health system payer.

Table 4
What can HTA agencies do to improve engagement with patients?

Summary of Main Findings
HTA agencies: 1. should have lay members on the board in sufficient numbers to have real input. 2. should engage with patient organisations relevant to the particular HTA on all topics. 3. need to have staff whose job it is to engage with patients. 4. need to understand that engagement = partnership and mutual give-and-take but not all patient organisations are realistically able to sustain that. 5. should support systematic access to education or capacity-building to enable patient organisations to be able to move to engagement. 6. should make a systematic commitment to share best practice throughout Europe – via EUnetHTA? 7. need to be clearer about what they expect from patients – and realistic (most are not scientists) so avoid too technical or scientific questions.

4. Final recommendations

Concluding the workshop, co-chairs Dr Karen Facey, Alastair Kent and Andrea Rappagliosi summarised the main focus of the recommendations:

1. **Policies for patient engagement**: every HTA Agency should create a clear policy outlining how they will involve patients in the HTA process and how that process will take account of patients' perspectives. Examples of best practice in Europe and internationally (eg including Canada and Australia) should be used to generate minimum standards for involvement that can be adapted and replicated nationally and locally. This should include examples from other related fields, such as the European regulatory processes where patients and patients' organisations are involved in the risk/benefit assessment and actively participate in the definition of what constitutes value.
2. **Education:** patients must be educated to better understand the concepts underpinning HTA so they understand how to contribute evidence that provides added value to the process. Similarly, HTA decision-makers and clinicians need to be better educated about patients' real-life experiences in order to move beyond clinical and cost-effectiveness issues when making decisions to take into account the full range of psychosocial aspects affecting patients' treatment and care: family and carer support, quality of life and wellbeing, employment etc.
3. **Resources:** increasing patient engagement will take manpower and resources and should be transparent (educational and financial support to patients' groups in order for them to participate, extra manpower at HTA agencies to help patients participate).
4. **Collaboration:** the only way to achieve real patient engagement in HTA is through greater collaboration between patients, HTA agencies, clinicians, academia and industry and to be clear about where and how collaboration can take place.

5. Next steps

The recommendations have been incorporated into the new Advanced Innovation Programme on HTA which was launched by Epposi in July 2011 taking account of the outcomes of further focus groups of HTA experts and wider consultation with all stakeholders between February and May 2011.

What has increasingly become apparent from these follow-up sessions is the need for wider societal needs and benefits to be included in HTAs, to go beyond narrow cost-effectiveness and efficacy parameters, and for education and training for *all* stakeholder groups – clinicians, patients, payers, industry, researchers, health economists, employers, politicians, policy-makers, regulators and HTA agency staff

– on how best to interact with one another and the HTA body from the start of an assessment process, in order to ensure the full impact is taken into account and reflected in better decision-making and outcomes.

As a non-advocacy organisation at a European level, Epposi members and stakeholders are well aware of the gaps in knowledge and ability to make themselves heard within the current systems of HTA around Europe. Epposi is currently finalising the scope of the research, which will incorporate current best practices and practical frameworks for implementation from across Europe. The programme will also focus on how the research can be applied to concrete skills enhancement throughout the process.

3. Physician perspectives

Pharmaceuticals Policy and Law 13 (2011) 205–212
DOI 10.3233/PPL-2011-0325
IOS Press

HTAs and access to rare diseases therapies: How can clinicians assist in the healthcare assessment of treatments for patients with primary immune deficiencies?

Helen Chapel[a,b]
[a]*Professor of Clinical Immunology, University of Oxford, Oxford, UK*
[b]*Department of Medicine, John Radcliffe Hospital, Oxford, UK*
E-mail: helen.chapel@ndm.ox.ac.uk

1. Background

Health Technology Assessments (HTA) in terms of therapies depend on established treatments for defined conditions with proven outcomes; the various treatment regimes can be compared with each other or with outcomes in the absence of treatment, in various healthcare settings. For example in the UK, the National Institute for Health Research – NIHR states that "The HTA programme produces independent research about the effectiveness of different healthcare treatments . . . for those who use, manage and provide care in the NHS".

Given limited financial resources, it is appropriate that HTA agencies are increasingly involved in assessment of the cost effectiveness of well -established therapies, including those for rare diseases. Ultimately HTAs are mechanisms that help funders and governments to control healthcare budget expenditure. An excellent example is the recent decision of the Irish Authority's Health Technology Assessment Directorate "not to introduce a new technology to screen donated blood for Creutzfeldt-Jakob disease because it would not be cost effective to do so". Such tools are widely used, though for rare diseases the background is often poorly understood. However their popularity is exemplified in the Journal Citation Reports for 2009, which shows that "Health Technology Assessment", the journal of the HTA programme, has seen a significant rise in its impact factor rising from 5.01 last year, to 6.91.

In the current world-wide economic climate, clinicians, patients, healthcare providers and those with the budgets need to understand the economic strategy of HTAs. This is particularly true for those involved with rare diseases, such as primary immune deficiencies (PIDs), and applies in countries with good access to PID centres of excellence that may be at risk, as well as in those in which therapies are restricted for financial reasons.

The role of HTAs in assessing the efficacy and cost effectiveness treatments for patients with PIDs is difficult for a variety of reasons: difficulties in setting up clinical trials in rare conditions, particularly when there is only one effective therapy; lack of long-term outcome data in recently recognized conditions; the lack of support for observational studies to collect data on a national or international basis. To this end, clinicians and others need to collaborate to collect increasing amounts of validated data in agreed formats, so that large numbers of PID patients – often from several EU countries – can be pooled for meaningful analysis and then interpreted for healthcare providers, who are keen to fund good medicine though not necessarily luxurious services. This is important for all but particularly for the recent EU accession countries where there needs to be wider availability of PID therapies. There is a growing appreciation of the financial and social implications of undiagnosed, and therefore untreated, PIDs but this needs to be underpinned by evidence-based data to ensure funding.

I will try to give a physician's eye view, to cover what we know and what we don't know in terms of currently established treatments for the various PID conditions that have proven outcomes, both with treatment and in the absence of treatment.

2. Primary Immune Deficiencies [PIDs]

The most important aspect of PIDs is the life-long nature of these diseases; the immune system, once defective, does not recover spontaneously but persists in failing to respond to infective organisms. This results in life-long susceptibility to severe, life-threatening or repeated infections. Many PID patients occur in infancy or childhood, often after several admissions to the ITU with severe infections. These types of PIDs are due to extensive failure of the immune system in which several types of immune cells are defective (Fig. 1). These defects are due to faulty genes, which can be passed to future generations or further siblings. In later life, the commonest forms of PIDs present from late adolescence to late middle age; patients suffer recurrent infections such as pneumonia or severe gastro-intestinal infections resulting in malabsorption. Like many chronic diseases, such as diabetes, these forms of PIDs probably result from a combination of several genes contributing to genetic susceptibility as well as unknown environmental triggers.

3. Range of PID diseases and severity

PIDs vary in severity depending on the extent of immune failure. Good, efficient immune responses are crucial for survival of all living things and it is not surprising that these responses involve at least 20 types of cells within at least 5 major categories. Genetic changes within any of these cells may result in reduced responses to infective organisms and so infections. This year the IUIS Expert PID committee listed 171 known diseases in which mutations in a single gene resulted in a PID and yet there will be many more once the "late onset" diseases are unraveled.

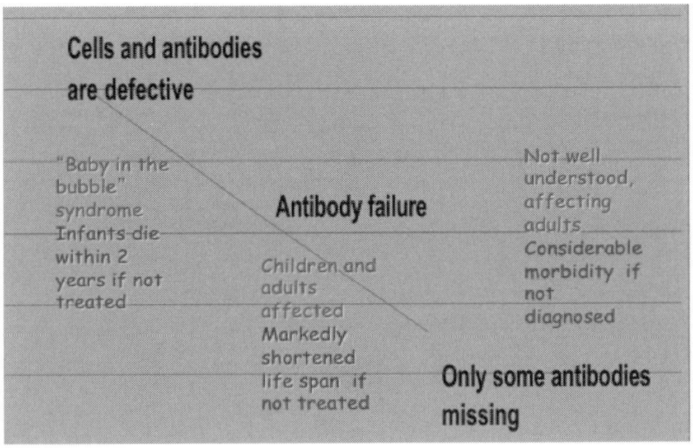

Fig. 1. Failure of immune components defines severity of disease. (Colours are visible in the online version of the article; http://dx.doi.org/10.3233/PPL-2011-0325)

4. PIDs are new and rare diseases

These are recent diseases, in that the first case of an immune deficiency was described in 1956. PIDs were only recognized as a particular group of diseases in the 1960s [5] (Fig. 2). This is not surprising since before the advent of antibiotics, those individuals with defective immune systems would have died of common infections without an underlying cause even being considered (Fig. 2). Once immunization against common infections became routine, individuals with preventable infections who had "failed" immunization, such as against polio, were recognized. Studies of patients with intrinsic immune defects, in whom there was no explanation for a severe or recurrent infections, began and the first series were published [3,5].

The prevalences of these conditions results in them being defined as "rare diseases", though the commonest symptomatic forms occur in 1:10,000 of the general population in western Europe, despite an under-diagnosis rate of around 50%.

The variable nature of the defects depends on the extent of the immune failure. In patients in whom both cells and antibodies fail, the immune deficiency is severe and infants and children with Severe Combined Immune Deficiency die before their second birthday. Patients with defects in antibody production have a reduced life-span (Fig. 3), though this has improved steadily over the last 40 years with the increasing availability of replacement antibody therapy.

5. Types of treatment for each disease group and prognosis

There are two types of therapy for those with immune deficiency: Human Stem Cell Transplantation (HSCT), using cord blood or bone marrow from healthy donors as a source of stem cells, for those missing immune cells; replacement antibodies,

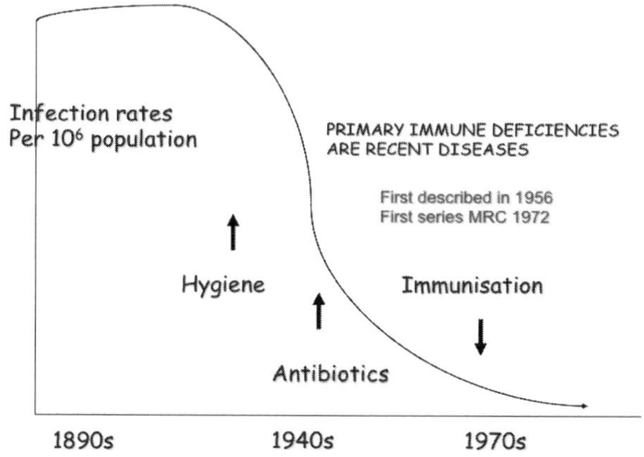

Fig. 2. Recognition of PID diseases in relation to medical advances. (Colours are visible in the online version of the article; http://dx.doi.org/10.3233/PPL-2011-0325)

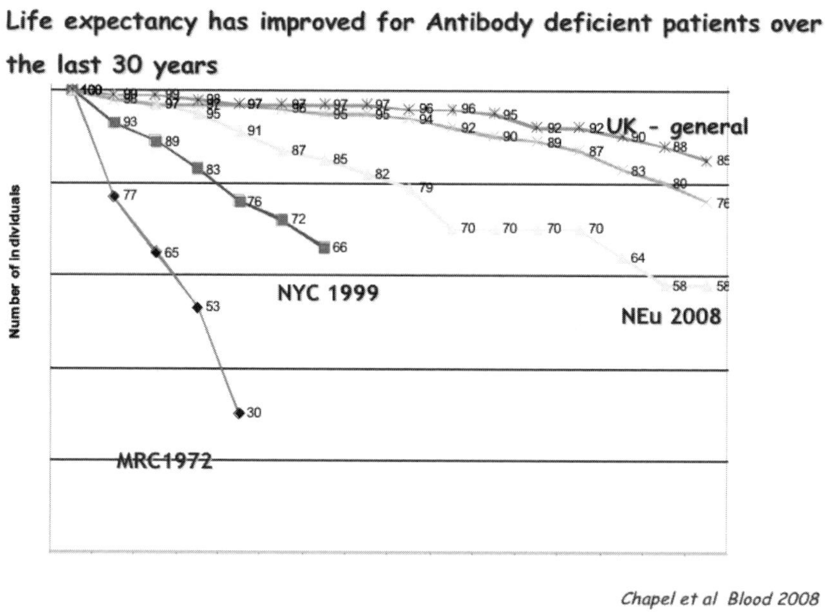

Fig. 3. Life expectancy has improved for Antibody Deficiency patients over the last 40 years. (Colours are visible in the online version of the article; http://dx.doi.org/10.3233/PPL-2011-0325)

known as therapeutic immunoglobulin (Ig) is used for those unable to produce their own antibodies. For Ig, blood is collected from normal donors and antibodies are purified. These therapies were not effective until the 1980s and remain the only treatments available. We know from the early series that the advent of such therapies has been life saving [5] (Fig. 3). First HSCT done with bone marrow from healthy donors (often relatives in early days till the crucial role of matching was appreciated) in the early 1970s. HSCT is now standard treatment now in many EU countries whose centres of excellence provide access to therapy for those outside their national boundaries and indeed outside the EU. However there is little pharmacoeconomic data as without replacement cells or antibodies, patients die of severe infections in infancy (Fig. 1). Clinical trials in severe PIDs are difficult due to the early age of patients and the huge variation in the types of these conditions depending on the defective immune gene concerned.

For those in whom only antibody production has failed, replacement therapeutic immunoglobulin (Ig) is available in many but not all EU countries without restriction for PID patients. To support this there have been some randomized clinical trials and data is now available as a meta-analysis. There has been a gradual improvement over the years in life expectancy [2]. Figure 3 – with increased availability of Ig in northern Europe. Unfortunately this improvement is not due to earlier diagnosis and therefore avoidance of complications, since diagnostic delay has not changed [9] – still more than 2 years for children and 4.5 years for adults.

6. Available data on therapy outcomes

Long-term observational studies are difficult to conduct but the data from a 25-year follow-up study [6] shows that severe infections can be prevented with adequate doses of Ig therapy though this is not the case in all EU countries due to restriction of supply [8]. In many EU states, governments put pressure on the PID community, either by making reimbursement increasingly difficult or by promoting lower treatment regimens. Fortunately the UK DoH understood these points and have exempt PIDs from Ig restrictions as there are no alternative therapies and effectiveness is proven [1] (Fig. 2).

The only approved therapies for severe immunodeficiencies are HSCT and Ig, though these are not available for patients in all EU member states. Although HSCT is curative, it is not without high risks of complications due to the increased life-threatening infection-risk until the new immune cells are established. In the future gene, therapy may be safer but the technology is still new and improved vectors for transferring normal copies of defective genes are being actively investigated.

7. Role of HTAs in PIDs

For diseases in which there are choices in terms of therapies, HTAs make sense. For example, the Swedish HTA agency is conducting an assessment of haemophilia prophylaxis treatment versus "on-demand" treatment. Factor VIII.clotting agents can be used as therapeutic treatment to stop bleeding or used prophylactically to reduce the risk of bleeding in treatment in haemophilia.

This is not possible in PID patients. For antibody deficient patients, Igs provide the only effective prophylaxis for potentially life-threatening infections, since it is not safe to use antibiotics alone. As discussed above, infants and children with severe immunodeficiencies (Fig. 1) die before two years of age without replacement immune systems.

8. Other considerations

The cost of treatment should be put into perspective with the financial burden of recurrent severe infections and other complications that result from failure to recognize a PID. Furthermore low or inappropriate treatment levels have associated consequences, including high rates of serious or persistent infections resulting in hospitalization and/or days of missed education or work; these also have associated costs.

9. Further studies to assist HTAs

What can physicians do to provide the type of data that can be used in a HTA, particularly in EU countries where HSCT is unavailable or Ig therapy is restricted to younger patients only? Physicians, including paediatricians, should focus on collecting evidence-based data on a long-term basis. This is probably best done in national registries, in order to collect data on appropriate selection of patients for therapies, determination of risk factors or prognostic indicators and criteria for various doses. Data can also be collected on complications such as bronchiectasis and surrogate markers for the morbidity.

Such registries are similar to those available for many common chronic, life-long diseases with expensive therapies. The best example is that of services for patients with chronic renal failure: of treatment opportunities for these patients include replacement filtration (dialysis) and replacement kidneys (transplantation), and decisions about appropriate therapy are made based on long-standing observational studies over 40 years on data collected by means of registries, both national and international enabling comparisons to be made between different types of services.

The types of data to be used in HTAs includes both qualitative and quantitative data. Physicians are used to collecting quantitative data but are less familiar with quality of life studies and do not necessarily have the skills to undertake them. We rely on epidemiologists and social scientists to help with these studies and rare diseases, such as PIDs, are not seen as a priority. There is also a much needed perspective to be achieved between best possible practice and reality; Murphy et al. put this well in an article in Health Technology Assessment [7] "Qualitative research is particularly useful to policy makers and planners by providing descriptive information and understanding of the context in which policies will be implemented".

10. Stakeholders

Fortunately there are EU initiatives that seek to involve key stakeholders, including physicians, social scientists and patient organisations such as the International Patient Organisiaton for Primary Immunodeficiencies (IPOPI) into the HTA process. The physicians on the International Union of Immunological Societies Expert committee for Primary Immune Deficiencies are concerned for wider access for treatment for PIDs in all countries and are willing to input into national HTAs and other assessments for either HSCT or Ig replacement therapies for PIDs. This committee (http://www.iuisonline.org/pages/primimmun.htm) worked with IPOPI to ensure that Ig therapy was included in the WHO Essential Medicines Lists, since at present this is the only treatment available for many PIDs. Now the focus is on removal of the restriction of this treatment in some countries to children or young adults despite inclusion in WHO Essential Medicines List for adult patients; since PIDs are life-long conditions, what happens to these young persons when they grow up if treatment is discontinued as in some EU countries at present?

11. World-wide sharing

The recently published Dublin Consensus statement comments particularly on the sharing of blood and blood products in view of the scarcity of plasma resources. "Blood components, plasma and plasma intermediates ... should be made available to meet the health needs of others and to contribute to global health outcomes". This should help to provide additional starting blood and plasma for the manufacture of therapeutic immunoglobulin in countries where availability is currently restricted.

In terms of ensuring that these scarce resources are widely available and used appropriately, the International Union of Immunological Societies (IUIS) Committee on PID produces advice on classification of immune deficiencies based on severity of disease, on a regular basis. International guidelines for diagnosis have been produced [4] and national organizations are actively involved in management guidelines [10,11].

12. Conclusions

In summary physicians can support appropriate treatment levels for PID patients by demonstrating the benefits early diagnosis and adequate treatment levels by setting up long-term outcome studies; observational databases are crucial. The success of the National Immunoglobulin Usage Guidelines in the UK shows that willingness of healthcare professionals to be involved as key stakeholders is important for healthcare providers too and since setting up home therapy programme registers in the UK and Europe, we know that treated patients have active working lives, contributing as tax payers and benefiting society in many other ways.

References

[1] H. Chapel and C. Cunningham-Rundles, Update in understanding common variable immunodeficiency disorders (CVIDs) and the management of patients with these conditions, *BJH* **145** (2009), 709–727.

[2] M. Chapel, M. Lucas, M. Lee, J. Bjorkander, D. Webster, B. Grimbacher, C. Fieschi, V. Thon, M.R. Abedi and L. Hammarstrom, Common variable immunodeficiency disorders: division into distinct clinical phenotypes, *Blood* **112** (2008), 277–286.

[3] M. Cooper, P.W. Faulk, H.H. Fudenberg, W. Hitzig, R.A. Good, H. Kunkel, F.S. Rosen, M. Seligmann, J. Soothill and R.J. Wedgwood, Classification of Primary Immunodeficiencies, *N Engl J Med* **288** (1973), 966–967.

[4] R. Geha, L.D. Notarangelo, J.L. Casanova, H. Chapel, M.E. Conley, A. Fischer, L. Hammarström, S. Nonoyama, H.D. Ochs, J.M. Puck, C. Roifman, R. Seger and J. Wedgwood, International Union of Immunological Societies Primary Immunodeficiency Diseases Classification Committee. Primary immunodeficiency diseases: an update from the International Union of Immunological Societies Primary Immunodeficiency Diseases Classification Committee, *J Allergy Clin Immunol* **120** (2007), 776–794.

[5] M. Healy, For the Medical Research Council working party on hypogammaglobulinaemia, Hypogammaglobulinaemia in the United Kingdom: XII Statistical analyses: prevalence, mortality and effects of treatment, *Special report series of the Medical Research Council (GB)* **310** (1971), 115–123.

[6] M. Lucas, M. Lee, J. Lortan, E. Lopez-Granados, S. Misbah and H. Chapel, Infection outcomes in patients with common variable immunodeficiency disorders: Relationship to immunoglobulin therapy over 22 years, *J Allergy Clin Immunol* **125** (2010), 1354–1360.

[7] E. Murphy, R. Dingwall, D. Greatbatch, S. Parker and P. Watson, Health Technology Assessment (2).

[8] I. Quinti, A. Soresina, A. Guerra, R. Rondelli, G. Spadaro, C. Agostini, C. Milito, A.C. Trombetta, V. Visentini, H. Martini, A. Plebani and M. Fiorilli, IPINet Investigators, Effectiveness of Immunoglobulin Replacement Therapy on Clinical Outcome in Patients with Primary Antibody Deficiencies: Results from a Multicenter Prospective Cohort Study, *J Clin Immunology* **31** (2011), 315–322.

[9] B. Seymour, J. Miles and M. Haeney, Primary antibody deficiency and diagnostic delay, *J Clin Path* **58** (2005), 546–547.

[10] M. Tang, Consensus recommendations for the use of immunoglobulin replacement therapy in immune deficiency. 1st Edition November 2008. Retrieved 29th June, 2009, from http://www.apiieg.org/STATEMENTS.ASP.

[11] P. Wood, S. Stanworth, J. Burton, A. Jones, D.G. Peckham, T. Green, C. Hyde and H. Chapel, Recognition, clinical diagnosis and management of patients with primary antibody defciencies: a systematic review, *Clin Exp Immunol* (2007).

Pharmaceuticals Policy and Law 13 (2011) 213–220
DOI 10.3233/PPL-2011-0326
IOS Press

What is the evidence produced so far by the application of HTA to haemophilia care?

Karin Berger*, Dorothee Schopohl and Wolfgang Schramm
Department of Transfusion Medicine and Hemostasis, University Hospital of Munich, Munich, Germany

1. Health Technology Assessment (HTA) – Importance in times of scarce resources

In times of escalating budget pressures the influence of payers and budget holders continues to increase. At the same time physicians are more and more limited prescribing expensive drugs. In the case of prescribing cost intensive therapies physicians are increasingly requested to justify their decision based on high clinical evidence. This changing health care environment has led to a rising need to demonstrate health outcomes in clinical research and under real life conditions. Health Technology Assessments (HTA) and Value Dossiers gain in importance to achieve reimbursement of therapies.

The main goal of HTA is determining the benefit of a health care technology on the basis of published clinical trials chosen from systematic literature searches and analyses [1]. Endpoints in the trials have to be clearly defined primary and secondary clinical outcomes for example "myocardial infarction" and not surrogate parameters as in this case "blood pressure". On the basis of outcomes in clinical trials, and information on costs, risks and benefits, which means weighting positive outcomes against frequency of adverse events to evaluate the resulting benefit of the health technology, a HTA can support decision-making. A HTA should provide information and transparency concerning the following aspects of a considered health technology: efficacy, real-life effectiveness, comparative effectiveness, health economic efficiency, and social, legal and ethical implications [2].

Concerning rare diseases, HTAs face specific problems regarding the availability of trials in general, very restricted patient numbers included in single trials, as well as ethical problems making randomization often impossible once a treatment or relief of symptoms has been found at all. The nature of rare diseases is usually chronic and

*Corresponding author: Karin Berger, Department of Transfusion Medicine and Hemostasis, University Hospital of Munich, Marchioninistrasse 15, D-81377 Munchen, Germany. Tel.: +49 89 5160 7434; Fax: +49 89 7095 8896; E-mail: Karin.Berger@med.uni-muenchen.de.

requires not only the inclusion of clinical outcomes like symptoms, complications and therapeutic adverse events, but also the consideration of patient-rated outcomes (PROs) like health-related quality of life, patients preferences/utilities, and activities and participation in normal life. Costs are usually considerable, and PROs can often only be measured after development of specialized clinimetric instruments.

2. Haemophilia – Outcomes research in a rare disease

2.1. Haemophilia – A rare disease

The prevalence of haemophilia A is 12.8 ± 6.0 (mean ± SD) for high income countries and 6.6 ± 4.8 per 100,000 males for the rest of the world [3], whereby Haemophilia A and haemophilia B occur with a ratio of approximately 4:1 [4]. Therefore haemophilia is a rare disease according to the definition of the European Union (EU) [affecting no more than 5 per 10,000 persons in the EU] [5]. Haemophilia is also a chronic, congenital disorder that requires lifelong replacement of the deficient clotting factors VIII or IX minimum during bleeding episodes [6]. Especially susceptible to bleeding in haemophilia are the joints, knees, ankles and elbows, whereby so-called target joints develop after repeated bleeding episodes into one joint leading to painful limitation of range of motion, and without treatment finally to crippling arthropathy [7]. Treatment of haemophilia consists of clotting factor replacement either as on-demand therapy after on-going bleeds only, or as prophylactic therapy with continuous factor substitution especially given in children to prevent bleeding episodes [8]. Whereas cost assessment is relatively simple in haemophilia due to the fact that approximately 90% of treatment costs are driven by factor concentrate, defined standardized outcome measures are all the more important to demonstrate evidence of therapeutic benefits.

2.2. Outcomes in haemophilia – Treatment benefits

Clinical health outcomes in haemophilia are primarily numbers of bleeding episodes, joint bleeds, and severe or life-threatening bleeds during defined periods of time and under defined treatment schedules with clotting factor concentrate. Joint damage caused by the repeated bleeding episodes is the next most frequently reported health outcome. Arthropathy can be measured by joint scores like the World Federation Orthopaedic Joint Score, the Haemophilia Joint Health Score (HJHS), the radiological Petterson score or the magnetic resonance imaging (MRI) joint score [4, 9]. The use of a variety of joint scores leads to a lack of standardization and accordance in the existing few trials. In addition, the inclusion of acute symptoms like pain and swelling, as well as chronic symptoms like limitation of range of motion in joint scores can lead to difficulties, if permanent deterioration must be rated separately from acute deterioration [10]. The same situation of lack of standardization and appropriate measurement instruments was found when health-related quality of life was evaluated in haemophilia patients in the past. Different instruments have been developed recently and validated for various countries [11], so that standardized application during trials is now possible [12].

To determine correlations between health outcome parameters like frequency of bleeding and joint scores [9], as well as joint scores and quality of life or degree of disability is still under development [13,14]. The International Haemophilia Prophylaxis Study Group tried to correlate the HJHS score with a self-report measure of physical disability, the modified Child Health Assessment Questionnaire (C-HAQmod), to the activity level of the children examined during validation of this paediatric joint scoring system [14]. The correlation failed because the C-HAQmod is predominantly weighted toward upper extremity tasks and not specific to detect discreet alterations in activity directed to tasks for lower extremities as to be expected in children with haemophilia from developed countries. Whereas the HJHS score is sensitive for mild arthropathy, correlation to and prediction of disability remains to be established.

A comprehensive analysis of treatment effects in a HTA is only possible if detailed information on clinical outcomes, as well as PROs is given in trials. In haemophilia care this comprises clinical endpoints like bleeding frequency, pain scores, radiologic joint scores, orthopedic joint scores, quality of life, clotting factor concentrate levels, time loss to school or employment, integration into society, well-being and global functioning [15]. Even so registries exist for haemophilia patients in various countries a major problem besides participation of physicians and collection of data from a sufficient patient number is quality and standardization of outcome data. Randomization of haemophilia patients is difficult not only because of low patient numbers, but especially because of ethical reasons. General requirements of HTAs to give detailed outcome information on specific health care products, i.e. different clotting factor preparations, can hardly be fulfilled. After the acquired immunodeficiency syndrome (AIDS) epidemic a diversity of clotting factor products is regarded not only desirable, but essential to ensure safe supply in case of failure of one product.

3. Haemophilia – Evidence generated in the past

3.1. Evidence in guidelines

Numerous guidelines worldwide deal with the analysis of the evidence in haemophilia treatment. To give an impression on the current status of evidence in haemophilia therapy the indications for replacement therapy using factor concentrates according to the "Cross-sectional guidelines for therapy with blood components and plasma derivatives" published by the German medical association in the 4th revised edition are shown in Table 1 with the respective levels of evidence [16]. The only 1 A level of evidence which is generated by "randomized, controlled studies without methodological flaws with unambiguous results" [16] was obtained so far for the prophylactic treatment of children and adolescents with severe haemophilia (Table 1).

3.2. Evidence in HTAs

Searching the Cochrane Library for "haemophilia" yielded two relevant publications [15,17]. A review by Stobart et al. from 2005 is apparently out-dated in its statement on lack of evidence for decrease in the frequency of joint bleeds by prophylactic clotting factor treatment [15]. The implications for research in haemophilia are, however, still valid in several aspects. The authors state, that future randomized trials should address the question of efficacy, safety and effectiveness of prophylactic versus on-demand treatment, which is still valid for adults, further the question of optimal regimen, as well as the question of standardized outcome measures of efficacy [15]. The second publication compares recombinant Factor VIIa concentrate with plasma derived concentrates for the treatment of acute bleeding episodes in patients with haemophilia and inhibitors [17]. Even so no difference could be found in efficacy and risk of thromboembolic complications, the authors state, that other non-randomized evidence can be taken in account when treatment is chosen in clinical practice. This statement points to individualized treatment often necessary in rare diseases and to the experience of the treating physician. One critical point addressed in the implications for research in this article is the need to define commonly agreed objective outcome measures so that research results can be pooled and evidence for important issues can be accumulated [17].

3.3. Availability of meta-analyses

A PubMed literature search conducted in June 2011 with the search-term "haemophilia AND meta-analysis" resulted in 54 hits. Successive selection by title and abstract revealed 26 relevant articles, two publications in Spanish, one consensus recommendation, four reviews and a total of 19 meta-analyses in English. Thereof, eight articles dealt with the topic inhibitor, three with B-domain deleted Factor VIII, two with recombinant Factor VIII, one with central venous access devices, one with mutation frequencies, one with Hepatitis C, one with bone mineral density, one with clinical outcome of radiosynoviorthesis, and only one article with the topic of prophylactic treatment and factor consumption.

Prospective randomized trials which can be combined to meta-analyses are generally scarce in rare diseases. The specialty of haemophilia is, that clinical outcome is mainly influenced by treatment pattern, i.e. on-demand or prophylaxis, and that treatment depends largely on the economic situation of a country [18]. In addition, haemophilia patients need individual tailored care, which is also typical for many rare diseases, but even more prominent in haemophilia due to individual half-lives of clotting factor in single patients and during a life-time [19]. Therefore the comparison of mean values may lead to wrong interpretations and may not be applicable to the situation of an individual patient.

3.4. Availability of cost analyses

A PubMed literature search conducted with the Medical Subjects Headings search-terms "costs" and "cost analysis" each combined with "hemophilia A" OR "hemophilia B" showed 43 cost studies between 1997 and 2008. The cost analyses on haemophilia treatment were mainly based on retrospective study designs, whereby 11 were studies with less than 100 patients, 2 were studies with more than 100 patients, 6 were multicenter studies with less than 100 patients, 13 were multicenter studies with more than 100 patients and 11 were studies focusing on special patient groups like patients undergoing surgery.

Prospective well conducted studies on economic issues in haemophilia are scarce. Most papers that have been written regarding the economics of prophylaxis in hemophilia consist of review and opinion papers. Many of these papers present interesting view points and summarize the minimal data that does exist on the economic evaluation of prophylaxis. Papers that contain primary data use different methodologies: retrospective, prospective, modeling, decision trees. In evaluating the outcomes of prophylaxis most papers have applied a cost-effectiveness strategy where the outcome represents a specific clinical measure, usually the number of joint bleeds. Using this measure of effectiveness most studies describe the incremental cost effectiveness ratio (ICER) as the incremental cost per joint bleed avoided. They do not present cost per quality adjusted life year what would make a comparison with other diseases possible, neither do they present budget impact figures.

4. Haemophilia – Evidence needed in the future

Comprehensive HTAs in haemophilia would have to consider bleeding frequency the degree of arthropathy and disability, the health-related quality of life and cost from a payer and a societal perspective. HTAs like this are not available because of the above mentioned specific features of haemophilia care, individualized therapy, ethical considerations and low patient numbers. In rare diseases evidence is often relying on small studies or case control studies, and even preparation of meta-analyses from small studies can be difficult because of lack of standardization and heterogeneous patient populations. Accordingly, also the preparation of recommendations and guidelines for rare diseases is limited due to lack of evidence as outlined in a report by the German Institute for Quality and Efficiency in Health Care (IQWIG). The only recommendation given so far is to investigate in observational studies, summing-up of small studies, and encouraging single case studies [20]. Nevertheless, researchers will have the duty to generate evidence as far as possible also for rare diseases. The recommendations of the second Wildbad Kreuth Meeting held in 2009 support this aim by the following two statements: (125) Registers of patients with haemophilia and related disorders should be established and maintained in each country. (133) Data on outcome of treatment should be collected, including clinical data such as

Table 1
Implications for replacement therapy using factor concentrates modified according to the "Cross-sectional guidelines for therapy with blood components and plasma derivatives" published by the German medical association in the 4th revised edition [16, page 86]

Treatment Principles	Overall assessment; classification	Assessment of the methodological validity of the underlying data; Implications
Factor replacement on demand shall be performed during spontaneous or traumatic bleeding episodes at any bleeding site if the bleeding exceeds a minimum degree (e.g. minor skin bleeding) [23,24].	**1 C+**	No randomized, controlled studies, but unambiguous data available. **Strong recommendation**
Full-time prophylactic replacement therapy shall be carried out mostly in **children and adolescents** with severe hemophilia in the form of physician-controlled self-administered treatment with the main intention of preventing hemophilic arthropathy [25–30].	**1 A**	Randomized, controlled studies without essential methodological flaws with unambiguous results. **Strong recommendation**
Full-time prophylactic replacement therapy can be carried out individually in **adults** with the intention of preventing the development of arthropathies as a late consequence [25,31–33].	**2 C+**	No randomized, controlled studies, but data can be extrapolated from other studies. **Weak recommendation**
Prophylactic therapy to prevent bleeding shall be provided before and after surgical interventions.	**1 C+**	No randomized, controlled studies, but unambiguous data available. **Strong recommendation**
Temporary prophylactic therapy to prevent bleeding should be provided during periods of major physical or psychic stress (e.g. rehabilitation, exams) [34,35].	**1 C**	Observational studies without control group, but with convincing results. **Medium strong recommendation**

frequency of bleedings and assessment of joint function as well as quality of life and economic information [21]. Recent accomplishment of randomized trials over many years to assess long-term effects of on-demand and prophylactic therapy in paediatric [22] and adult haemophilia patients [12] encourages and confirms the efforts already made to obtain evidence, to optimize therapy and in the long run also to save costs.

References

[1] C. Brettschneider, D. Luhmann and H. Raspe, Informative value of Patient Reported Outcomes (PRO) in Health Technology Assessment (HTA), *GMS Health Technol Assess* **7** (2011), Doc01.

[2] B. O'Mahony, D. Noone and K. Tolley, An Introduction to Key Concepts in Health Economics for Hemophilia Organizations, *Hemophilia Organization Development* (2010), 1–22.

[3] J.S. Stonebraker, P.H. Bolton-Maggs, J.M. Soucie, I. Walker and M. Brooker, A study of variations in the reported haemophilia A prevalence around the world, *Haemophilia* **16** (2010), 20–32.

[4] B.M. Feldman, S. Funk, B. Lundin, A.S. Doria, R. Ljung and V. Blanchette, Musculoskeletal measurement tools from the International Prophylaxis Study Group (IPSG), *Haemophilia* **14**(Suppl 3) (2008), 162–169.

[5] Commission, of, the, European, Communities. Communication from the Commission of the European Parliament, the Council, the European Economic and Social Committee and the Committee of the Regions on Rare Diseases: Europe's challenges {SEC(2008)2713} {SEC(2008)2712}. Brussels, 11.11.2008.

[6] R. Ljung, Prophylactic therapy in haemophilia, *Blood Rev* **23** (2009), 267–274.

[7] L.A. Valentino, Controversies regarding the prophylactic management of adults with severe haemophilia A, *Haemophilia* **15**(Suppl 2) (2009), 5–18, quiz 9–22.

[8] W. Schramm, S. Royal, B. Kroner et al., Clinical outcomes and resource utilization associated with haemophilia care in Europe, *Haemophilia* **8** (2002), 33–43.

[9] K. Fischer, B.A. van Hout, J.G. van der Bom, D.E. Grobbee and H.M. van den Berg, Association between joint bleeds and Pettersson scores in severe haemophilia, *Acta Radiol* **43** (2002), 528–532.

[10] P. Collins, A. Faradji, M. Morfini, M.M. Enriquez and L. Schwartz, Efficacy and safety of secondary prophylactic vs. on-demand sucrose-formulated recombinant factor VIII treatment in adults with severe hemophilia A: results from a 13-month crossover study, *J Thromb Haemost* **8** (2010), 83–89.

[11] M. Bullinger, D. Globe, J. Wasserman, N.L. Young and S. von Mackensen, Challenges of patient-reported outcome assessment in hemophilia care-a state of the art review, *Value Health* **12** (2009), 808–820.

[12] A. Tagliaferri, G. Rivolta, A. Coppola et al., Prophylaxis versus on-demand therapy through economic report (P.O.T.T.E.R.) study, *J Thromb Haemost* **7** (2009), 819.

[13] K. Fischer, J.G. Bom, E.P. Mauser-Bunschoten, G. Roosendaal and H.M. Berg, Effects of haemophilic arthropathy on health-related quality of life and socio-economic parameters, *Haemophilia* **11** (2005), 43–48.

[14] B.M. Feldman, S.M. Funk, B.M. Bergstrom et al., Validation of a new pediatric joint scoring system from the International Hemophilia Prophylaxis Study Group: validity of the hemophilia joint health score, *Arthritis Care Res (Hoboken)* **63** (2011), 223–230.

[15] K. Stobart, A. Iorio and J.K. Wu, Clotting factor concentrates given to prevent bleeding and bleeding-related complications in people with hemophilia A or B, *Cochrane Database Syst Rev* (2005), CD003429.

[16] Bundesärztekammer, (German, Medical, Association). Cross-sectional Guidelines for Therapy with Blood Components and Plasma Derivatives; 4th revised edition. 2009.

[17] A. Iorio, D. Matino, R. D'Amico and M. Makris, Recombinant Factor VIIa concentrate versus plasma derived concentrates for the treatment of acute bleeding episodes in people with haemophilia and inhibitors, *Cochrane Database Syst Rev* (2010), CD004449.

[18] J.S. Stonebraker, M. Brooker, R.E. Amand, A. Farrugia and A. Srivastava, A study of reported factor VIII use around the world, *Haemophilia* **16** (2010), 33–46.

[19] V.S. Blanchette, Prophylaxis in the haemophilia population, *Haemophilia* **16**(Suppl 5) (2010), 181–188.

[20] Welche Evidenz wird für die Erstellung von Leitlinien für seltene Erkrankungen derzeit herangezogen? (Rapid Report). *IQWIG-Berichte*. Köln: Institut für Qualität und Wirtschaftlichkeit im Gesundheitswesen (IQWIG; Institute for Quality and Efficiency in Health Care) Bundesministerium für Gesundheit (Federal Ministry of Health); ISSN: 1864-2500, 2011 Nr. 83.

[21] Optimal clinical Use of Blood Components (Proceedings). Wildbad Kreuth, Bavaria, Germany: International Symposium co-organized by the EDQM & HealthCare/DBO – Transfusion Medicine, council of Europe, PEI, the German Official National Agency for Biologicals, The Transfusionsmedizin und Haemostasologie , Klinikum der Universitaet Muenchen; ISBN 978-3-86853-674-4, 24–25 April 2009.

[22] A. Gringeri, B. Lundin, S. von Mackensen, L. Mantovani and P.M. Mannucci, A randomized clinical trial of prophylaxis in children with hemophilia A (the ESPRIT Study), *J Thromb Haemost* **9** (2011), 700–710.

[23] J.M. Lusher, C.A. Lee, C.M. Kessler and C.L. Bedrosian, The safety and efficacy of B-domain deleted recombinant factor VIII concentrate in patients with severe haemophilia A, *Haemophilia* **9** (2003), 38–49.

[24] K. Schimpf, B. Fischer and P. Rothmann, Hemophilia A prophylaxis with factor VIII concentrate in a home-treatment program: a controlled study, *Scand J Haematol Suppl* **30** (1977), 79–80.

[25] K. Fischer, J.G. van der Bom, P. Molho et al., Prophylactic versus on-demand treatment strategies for severe haemophilia: a comparison of costs and long-term outcome, *Haemophilia* **8** (2002), 745–752.

[26] R.A. Gruppo, D. Brown, M.M. Wilkes and R.J. Navickis, Comparative effectiveness of full-length and B-domain deleted factor VIII for prophylaxis – a meta-analysis, *Haemophilia* **9** (2003), 251–260.

[27] M.J. Manco-Johnson, T.C. Abshire, A.D. Shapiro et al., Prophylaxis versus episodic treatment to prevent joint disease in boys with severe hemophilia, *N Engl J Med* **357** (2007), 535–544.

[28] S. Royal, W. Schramm, E. Berntorp et al., Quality-of-life differences between prophylactic and on-demand factor replacement therapy in European haemophilia patients, *Haemophilia* **8** (2002), 44–50.

[29] K. Steen Carlsson, S. Hojgard, A. Glomstein et al., On-demand vs. prophylactic treatment for severe haemophilia in Norway and Sweden: differences in treatment characteristics and outcome, *Haemophilia* **9** (2003), 555–566.

[30] H.M. van den Berg, K. Fischer, J.G. van der Bom, G. Roosendaal and E.P. Mauser-Bunschoten, Effects of prophylactic treatment regimens in children with severe haemophilia: a comparison of different strategies, *Haemophilia* **8**(Suppl 2) (2002), 43–46.

[31] L.M. Aledort, R.H. Haschmeyer and H. Pettersson, A longitudinal study of orthopaedic outcomes for severe factor-VIII-deficient haemophiliacs. The Orthopaedic Outcome Study Group, *J Intern Med* **236** (1994), 391–399.

[32] M.D. Carcao and L. Aledort, Prophylactic factor replacement in hemophilia, *Blood Rev* **18** (2004), 101–113.

[33] I. Plug, J.G. van der Bom, M. Peters et al., Thirty years of hemophilia treatment in the Netherlands, 1972–2001, *Blood* **104** (2004), 3494–3500.

[34] W. Schramm. Deutsche Hämophiliegesellschaft (DHG) – Ärztlicher Beirat. Konsensus Empfehlungen zur Hämophiliebehandlung in Deutschland. 11. März 1993, *Haemostaseologie* **14** (1994), 81–83.

[35] W. Schramm and I. Scharrer, Konsensus Empfehlungen zur Hämophiliebehandlung in Deutschland. GTH Hämophiliekommission, update 1999, *Hämophilieblätter* **34** (2000), 62–65.

4. HTA Agency perspectives

Pharmaceuticals Policy and Law 13 (2011) 223–232
DOI 10.3233/PPL-2011-0327
IOS Press

Orphan drugs in oncology

Claudia Wild[a,*], Katharina Hintringer[a,b] and Anna Nachtnebel[a]
[a]*Ludwig Boltzmann Institute for Health Technology Assessment, Vienna, Austria*
[b]*Department of Public Health and Health Technology Assessment, Institute of Public Health, Medical Decision Making and Health Technology Assessment, University for Health Sciences, Medical Informatics and Technology, Tyrol, Austria*

1. Introduction

Since the EMA/ European Medicines Agency has implemented a regulation intending to stimulate the development of drugs for rare diseases in 2000, 858 drugs have received Orphan Drug Designations, but only 62 drugs have yet received Marketing Authorisation as an "orphan drug". To benefit from the incentives (reduced fees for marketing-authorisation applications and protection from market competition), companies intending to develop an orphan medicine must submit an application to the European Medicines Agency requesting 'orphan designation' for their medicine. The application is evaluated by the Agency's Committee for Orphan Medicinal Products (COMP), which provides its opinion on whether or not the medicine qualifies as an orphan medicine for the treatment, prevention or diagnosis of a rare disease, defined as a condition affecting no more than 5 in 10,000 people in the EU. If the COMP issues a positive opinion, the EMA may then grant the medicine orphan status: all of them registered in the Register of designated Orphan Medicinal Products [1].

Even though a wide variety of diseases fulfil this criterion, the largest group (45.2%) for which the COMP has adopted a positive opinion as well as of the 62 drugs finally having received marketing authorisation (35.5)% were for oncology treatments [2]. By April 2011, 21 oncologic drugs (between 1 and 5 per year) have been approved as orphan drugs (see Table 1), some of them for more than one indication. According to industry-forecasts, the number of designations will "continue to increase exponentially" [3] within the next months and years and consequently will the number of successful marketing authorisations.

While the regulation for orphan drugs, originally intended to provide a favourable economic environment for the development of drugs for which either no market or a too fragmented markets for the generation of adequate return on investment exist, is euphorically discussed in pharma-fora and at biotech-conferences, health

*Corresponding author: Claudia Wild, Ludwig Boltzmann Institute for Health Technology Assessment, Garnisongasse 7/20, 1090 Vienna, Austria. E-mail: Claudia.Wile@hta.lbg.ac.at.

Table 1

Approved orphan drugs in oncology indications

	Trade Name	Substance name	Licensed Indication(s)	Date of authorization	Extras	Prevalence / Indication	prevalence per 10,000 pop.	absolute number of pts affected EU wide
1	Afinitor	everolimus	Carcinoma, Renal Cell	03.08.2009		Renal cell carcionoma	4,2	193.000
2	Arzerra	ofatumumab	Leukemia, Lymphocytic, Chronic, B-Cell	19.04.2010	C	Chronic lymphocytic leukemia	3,5	176.000
3	Atriance	nelarabine	Precursor T-Cell Lymphoblastic Leukemia-Lymphoma	22.08.2007	E	Acute lymphoblastic Leukemia	1,1	51.000
4	Ceplene	histamine dihydrochloride	acute myeloid leukaemia (AML)	07.10.2008	E	Acute myeloid leukemia	0,7	32.000
5	Evoltra	clofarabine	Precursor Cell Lymphoblastic Leukemia-Lymphoma	29.05.2006	E	Acute lymphoblastic Leukemia	0,4	15.000
6	Gliolan	5-aminolevulinic acid hydrochloride	Glioma	07.09.2007		Gliomas	1,0	37.000
7 - 1	Glivec	imatinib	Leukemia, Myelogenous, Chronic, BCR-ABL Positive Dermatofibrosarcoma Gastrointestinal Stromal Tumors Hypereosinophilic Syndrome Myelodysplastic-Myeloproliferative Diseases Precursor Cell Lymphoblastic Leukemia-Lymphoma	07.11.2001		Malignant gastrointestinal stromal tumours	0,1	2.250
7 - 2						Acute lymphoblastic leukaemia	0,5	23.000
7 - 3						Chronic myeloid leukaemia	0,9	34.000
7 - 4						Myelodysplastic / myeloproliferative diseases	1,6	74.000
7 - 5						Dermatofibrosarcoma protuberans	1,0	46.000
7 - 6						Chronic eosinophilic leukaemia and the hypereosinophilic syndrome	1,0	46.000
8	Litak	cladribine	Leukemia, Hairy Cell	14.04.2004		Indolent non-Hodgkin's lymphoma	2,4 to 3, 65	90.000 to 138.000
9	Lysodren	mitotane	Adrenal Cortex Neoplasms	28.04.2004		Adrenocortical carcinoma	0,11	4.000
10	Mepact	mifamurtide	Osteosarcoma	06.03.2009		Osteosarcoma	0,5	19.000
11	Mozobil	plerixafor	Multiple Myeloma, Lymphoma: Hematopoietic Stem Cell Transplantation	31.07.2009		Mobilize progenitor cells prior to stem cell transplantation	less than 1	46.000
12 -1	Nexavar	sorafenib	Renal Cell Carcinoma Hepatocellular Carcinoma	19.07.2006		Renal Cell Carcinoma	3	116.000
12 - 2						Hepatocellular Carcinoma	1	46.000
13	Revlimid	lenalidomide	Multiple Myeloma	14.06.2007		Multiple Myeloma	1,3	50.000
14	Sprycel	dasatinib	Acute lymphoblastic leukaemia	20.11.2006		Acute lymphoblastic leukaemia	0,7	33.000
15	Sprycel	dasatinib	Chronic myeloid leukaemia	20.11.2006		Chronic myeloid leukaemia	0,9	41.000
16	Tasigna	nilotinib	Chronic myeloid leukaemia	19.11.2007		Chronic myeloid leukaemia	1	46.000
17	Thalidomide Celgene	thalidomide	Multiple Myeloma	16.04.2008		Multiple Myeloma	1,2	45.000
18 - 1	Torisel	temsirolimus	Renal Cell Carcinoma, Mantle-Cell Lymphoma	19.11.2007		Renal cell carcinoma	3,5	16.1000
18 - 2						Mantle-Cell Lymphoma	0,4	18.000
19	Trisenox	arsenic trioxide	Leukemia, Promyelocytic, Acute	05.03.2002		Acute promyelocytic leukaemia	0,8	30.000
20 - 1	Vidaza	azacitidine	Myelodysplastic Syndromes, acute myeloid leukaemia	17.12.2008		Myelodysplastic Syndromes	1,1 - to 3	41.000 – 113.000
20 - 2						Acute myeloid leukaemia	<2	<100.000
21- 1	Yondelis	trabectedin	Ovarian Neoplasms, Soft tissue sarcoma	17.09.2007	E	Ovarian Neoplasms	2,4	92.000
21- 2						Soft tissue sarcoma	0,6	23.000

E = exceptional circumstances
C = conditional approval

Table 2
Turnover of orphan drugs in oncology in Germany 2009 [27]

DRUG		Turnover in mio €
Trade Name	substance name	
Glivec	imatinib	262,60 Mio
Revlimid	lenalidomide	77,80 Mio
Nexavar	sorafenib	58,80 Mio
Afinitor	everolimus	20,50 Mio
Sprycel	dasatinib	18,90 Mio
Tasigna	nilotinib	16,70 Mio
Thalidomide Celgene	thalidomide	2,70 Mio
Vidaza	azacitidine	2,30 Mio
Torisel	temsirolimus	1,60 Mio

care researchers and politicians are increasingly concerned about the exploitation of the regulation. These concerns are twofold: the lack of evidence at the time of approval [4] and the staggered approvals for small indications, eventually resulting in a large number of potential patients [5,6].

For medicines already approved and available on the market, that can be additionally licensed for an orphan disease indication and therefore remarketed Imatinib (Glivec®) is often cited as an example: Imatinib is indicated for six separate rare malignancies and was gradually approved between 2001 and 2006. In Germany – as in other countries – Glivec® has become a blockbuster with 262.6 Mio turnover in 2009, ranking 6th in the list of top-sellers. Similar to Glivec®, 10% of all orphan drugs turned into blockbusters by definition (>1 billion US$ annual turnover) [7].

"A growing number of drugs are initially licensed for a small indication, or limited to a subset of patients within one narrowly defined pathology, even though their pharmacological activity suggests they could be useful for a wider target population and/or for a range of pathologies. Early access for those patients with a high unmet need is enabled on the basis of limited data, but with each additional (sub-) indication, new data, often from randomized controlled trials, contribute to the safety database, enabling a more refined benefit/risk assessment" [5]. Some call it loopholes in legislation [8], others exploitation for profit [9] or market abuse, but many raise the issue of an increasing need for consumer protection [10].

While orphan drug designation and market authorisation are activities and decisions taken at the level of the EU/European Union, drug reimbursement decisions are national decisions in individual member states based on national regulatory processes and national budgets available. Several countries have indicated that HTA/ health technology assessment is the method of choice, treating "orphan drugs as any other drug available" [11–14]. In Austria, embedded in the general LBI-HTA work program a Horizon Scanning Program for oncology drugs was launched in 2007 [15]. After refining the underlying methods, first assessments were conducted in October 2009.

2. Early assessments of (orphan) drugs in oncology

The Horizon Scanning System in Oncology/HSS-O aims at the early assessment of drugs shortly before/ after EMA approval or, at least, before the routine use in clinical practice comprising new anticancer drugs as well as already established anticancer drugs with a planned extension of indication [15]. Naturally, orphan drugs are among them, but no differentiation is made to other drugs without special status. Since the establishment of the HSS-O in October 2009, 17 Assessments about new anticancer drugs have been published by the LBI-HTA. Out of these drugs, 6 (35%) had an orphan drugs designation and were approved as orphan drugs in the indication of interest. These were:

- Azacitidine (Vidaza®) for the treatment of myelodysplastic syndromes [16]
- Everolimus (Afinitor®) for the treatment of renal cell carcinoma [17]
- Trabectedin (Yondelis®) for the treatment of ovarian cancer [18]
- Plerixafor (Mozobil®) for the treatment to mobilize progenitor cells prior to stem cell transplantation [19]
- Nilotinib (Tasigna®) for the treatment of chronic myeloid leukaemia [20]
- Dasatinib (Sprycel®) for the treatment of chronic myeloid leukaemia [21]

Azacitidine (Vidaza®): In December 2008, the EMA granted market authorization for Vidaza® for patients not eligible for bone marrow transplantation suffering from intermediate-2 and high risk myelodysplastic syndromes, for chronic myelomonocytic leukaemia with 10% to 29% marrow blasts without myeloproliferative disorders and for patients with acute myeloid leukaemia with 20% to 30% blasts and multi-lineage dysplasia. This decision was based on a study which demonstrated an improvement in overall survival by 9.5 months (HR = 0.58, $p = 0.0001$) for patients treated with azacitidine in comparison to three other regimens (best supportive care, low-dose cytarabine, intensive chemotherapy). A subgroup analysis of azacitidine in comparison to intensive chemotherapy showed lower rates of infections for the azacitidine group, but failed otherwise to demonstrate improved outcomes.

Everolimus (Afinitor®): About 2 years after everolimus had received the orphan drug designation, market authorization was granted for the treatment of patients with metastatic or advanced renal cell carcinoma after failure of treatment with sunitinib or sorafenib in August 2009. In a cross-over trial, progression-free survival was prolonged by 2.1 months in comparison to placebo (HR = 0.30). Even though everolimus was the first agent which demonstrated benefits for patients with renal cell carcinoma after tyrosine kinase inhibitor therapy, no improvements were found either for overall survival or for quality-of-life.

Trabectedin (Yondelis®): Trabectedin is an antineoplastic agent approved for the treatment of soft tissue sarcoma and for patients with relapsed/recurrent platinum-sensitive ovarian cancer (OC) in Europe. Whereas, EMA granted marketing authorisation in September 2009 for OC, the US Food and Drug Administration (US FDA) voted 14:1 against the approval of trabectedin due to concerns whether the benefit of

Table 3

Study details of 6 approved orphan drugs with oncological indications

Approval status for this indication

DSD Nr.	Report filed	Drug Name	Indication	ODD Indication	ODD year	EMA	FDA	Comparator (phase III trials)	Primary outcome(s) of fully published phase III trials (I vs C)	estimated monthly costs in € (if not otherwise indicated)	prevalence per 10,000 population	absolute number of pts affected EU wide	trial registry number of pivotal phase III trial	study design of pivotal phase III trial	duration of pivotal phase III study
DSD 01	Okt.09	Azacitidine (Vidaza ®)	myelodysplastic syndromes (MDS)	myelodysplastic syndromes	2002	Dez.08	Mai.04	active	_OS_ *(at median follow-up of 21.1 months):* 24.5 vs 15 months; HR=0.58 (95% CI 0.43 - 0.77; p=0.0001)	5,400.-	1,1 - 3	41.000 - 113.000	NCT00071799	multicenter, randomized, open-label, parallel-group	4 years (Nov 2003 - July 2007)
DSD 03	Okt.09	Everolimus (Afinitor ®)	advanced kidney cancer after failure of treatment with sunitinib or sorafenib	renal cell carcinoma	2007	Aug.09	Mär.09	placebo	_median PFS:_ 4.4 vs. 4.2 months; HR=0.90 (95% CI 0.76 - 1.00; p=0.24)	initial starting dose: 2,000 monthly costs of 3,900	4,20	193.000	NCT00410124	multicenter, randomized, double-blind, placebo-controlled	4.5 years (Oct 2006 - May 2011)
DSD 07	Jän.10	Trabectedin (Yondelis ®)	2nd-line recurrent platinum-sensitive ovarian cancer	ovarian cancer	2003	Sep.09	refusal of marketing authorization 07/2009	active	_median PFS:_ 7.3 vs 5.8 months; HR=0.79 (95% CI 0.65 - 0.96; p=0.02)	1 treatment cycle trabectedin (=3 weeks): 3,900	2,4	92.000	NCT00113607	multicenter, randomized, open-label	6 years (April 2005 - May 2011)
DSD 08	Apr.10	Plerixafor (Mozobil®)	autologous hematopoietic stem cell transplantation for lymphoma and multiple myeloma	for treatment to mobilze progenitor cells prior to stem cell transplantation	2004	Jul.09	Dez.09	placebo (2 studies)	_proportion of patients collecting CD34+ cells:_ 1st study: proportion of patients collecting ≥6 x 106 CD34+ cells/kg in ≤ 2 apharesis days: 71.6 %vs 34.4%; HR=2.54 (p<0.001) 2nd study: proportion of patients able to mobilize ≥5 x 106 CD34+ cells/kg in ≤ 4 apharesis days: 59.3% vs 19.6%; HR=3.64 (95% CI 2.39 - 5.45, p<0.0001)	Given to a maximum of four consecutive days: 6,600 - 26,600	<1	46.000	NCT00103662; NCT00103610	multicenter, randomized, double-blind, placebo-controlled; multicenter, randomized, double-blind, placebo-controlled, comparative trial	3 years (Jan 2005 - Jan 2008); 3 years (Jan 2005 - Dec 2007)

Table 3, continued

DSD Nr.	Report filed	Drug Name	Indication	ODD Indication	ODD year	EMA	FDA	Comparator (phase III trials)	Primary outcome(s) of fully published phase III trials (I vs C)	estimated monthly costs in € (if not otherwise indicated)	prevalence per 10,000 population	absolute number of pts affected EU wide	trial registry number of pivotal phase III trial	study design of pivotal phase III trial	duration of pivotal phase III study
DSD 15	Jän.11	Nilotinib (Tasigna ®)	1st-line therapy in patients with philadelphia-chomosome positive chronic myeloid leukaemia in the chronic phase (Ph+ CML-CP)	chronic myeloid leukaemia	2006	Dez.10	Jun.10	active (3 arms - I1: nilotinib 300mg twice daily, I2: nilotinib 400mg twice daily, C: imatinib 400mg once daily	_major molecular response at 12 months:_ 44% vs 43% vs 22% (p<0.001) _complete cytogenetic response at 12 months:_ 80% vs 78% vs 65% (p<0.0001)	not yet available in Austria	1	46.000	NCT00471497	multicenter, randomized, open-label	6 years (July 2007 - May 2013)
DSD 17	Apr.11	Dasatinib (Sprycel ®)	1st-line therapy in patients with philadelphia-chomosome positive chronic myeloid leukaemia in the chronic phase	chronic myeloid leukaemia	2005	Dez.10	Okt.10	active	_confirmed complete cytogenetic response at 12 months:_ 77% (95% CI 71 - 82) vs 66% (95% CI 60 - 72; p=0.007)	estimated: 4,450	0,9	41.000	NCT00481247	multicenter, randomized, open-label	6.5 years (Sept 2007 - Jan 2014)

the trabectedin therapy can outweigh its harm without demonstration of an increase in overall survival in the pivotal OVA-301 trial. The primary outcome PFS at an interim analysis of the OVA-301 trial within the overall study population was 7.3 (95% CI 5.9 to 7.9) months in the intervention group (pegylated liposomal doxorubicin PLD) followed by trabectedin) and 5.8 (95% CI 5.5 to 7.1) months within the control group (PLD alone) (HR = 0.79 (95% CI 0.65 to 0.96, $p = 0.019$).

Plerixafor (Mozobil®): Plerixafor is used in combination with G-CSF to mobilize haematopoietic stem cells (HSC) from the bone marrow into the peripheral blood and aims to decrease the number of aphaeresis sessions needed to collect a sufficient number of HSC for HSC transplantation (HSCT) in patients suffering from haematological malignancies eligible for HSCT compared to stem cell mobilization with G-CSF alone. In July, EMA approved plerixafor in combination with G-CSF for the mobilization of HSC in lymphoma and multiple myeloma (MM) patients whose cells mobilize poorly based on the results of 2 phase III trials assessing the safety and efficacy of plerixafor – one in patients with MM and one in patients with Non-Hodgkin's Lymphoma (NHL). The primary outcome in the MM trial was the proportion of patients collecting a certain number of CD34+ cells/kg in two or less aphaeresis days. 71.6% of the intervention group (G-CSF + plerixafor) and 34.4% in the control group (G-CSF + placebo) reached the primary endpoint ($p < 0.001$). Within the NHL trial 59.3% of the intervention group (G-CSF + plerixafor) and 19.6% within the control group (G-CSF + placebo) reached the primary outcome of collecting a certain amount of CD34+ cells/kg in four or less aphaeresis days ($p < 0.001$). Despite plerixafor is approved for patients who are considered to be poor mobilizers, the population included in the pivotal phase III trials were adequate or good mobilizers.

Nilotinib (Tasigna®): Nilotinib, a second-generation tyrosine kinase inhibitor (TKI) aims to significantly reduce proliferation of CML cells carrying a certain gene.The current standard of care for 1st-line therapy in patients with Philadelphia-chromosome positive chronic myeloid leukaemia in the chronic phase (Ph+ CML-CP) is imatinib mesylate. In November 2007, EMA approved nilotinib for a subgroup of CML patients who are intolerant to prior therapy including imatinib. Since December 2010 nilotinib is approved for the 1st-line therapy in Ph+ CML-CP patients based on interim (12-months' visit of the last patient randomized) safety and efficacy data of the pivotal phase III trial, ENESTnd. The aim of ENESTnd was to investigate two different dosing regimens of nilotinib (either nilotinib 300 mg twice daily or nilotinib 400 mg twice daily) compared to 400 mg imatinib. The primary outcome, major molecular response, was achieved by 44% in the nilotinib 300 mg group, 43% in the nilotinib 400 mg group and 22% in the control group.

Dasatinib (Sprycel®): Dasatinib is as Nilotinib, a second-generation TKI which aims as nilotinib to reduce proliferation CML cells. In 2006 EMA approved dasatinib for the treatment of CML-CP patients after failure of imatinib therapy. Since December 2010 dasatinib is also approved for the 1st-line therapy in this indication based on interim data of the DASISION trial (dasatinib 100 mg once daily vs. 400 mg imatinib once daily; 12-months follow-up visit of the last patient randomized). The primary outcome of the DASISION trial is the surrogate endpoint confirmed complete cytogenetic response by 12 months which is 77% (95% CI 71 to 82) and 66% (95% CI 60 to 72; $p = 0.007$) for the intervention and control group, respectively. Based on these interim results, both regulatory agencies – EMA and the US Food and Drug Administration (FDA) – granted marketing authorization for the 1st-line therapy of patients with Ph+ CML-CP provided, the marketing authorization holder committed to the post-marketing requirement to submit long-term follow-up data, at least 5 years, from the DASISION trial.

To summarize: Out of the six drugs assessed within our HSS-O, overall survival, still the gold-standard for the efficacy of oncologic drugs, was used as primary outcome measure only for azacitidine. The trials investigating trabectedin and everolimus evaluated the drugs' impact on progression-free survival (PFS). Everolimus prolonged PFS in comparison to placebo by 2.2 months, but no differences emerged for OS, possibly due to the cross-over design of that trial. PFS differed between trabectedin and another active substance by 1.5 months, but no results are available for OS. The remaining 3 drugs which were subject of our assessments were licensed based on surrogate parameters only, including molecular response and cytogenetic response or number of CD34+ cells. The monthly costs for these drugs ranged from about € 4,000 to € 5,400.

3. Summary and conclusion

Despite the industry's claim that the demonstration of added clinical value is a "challenge", because of the low prevalence of rare diseases entailing low statistical power to detect significant effects on clinical outcome measures, there is a strong and outspoken agreement among the HTA-agencies that orphan drugs have to prove effectiveness like any other drug before their broad introduction into clinical practice and/or public reimbursement [11–14]. Another concern is that reimbursement decisions are not only based on effectiveness analysis, but also on cost-effectiveness considerations, but many orphan drugs tend to fail threshold criteria, because the costs for orphan drug treatments are usually higher than for many non-rare-disease treatments.

As a consequence of this gap between lack of proven effectiveness at the time of approval and enormous prices for new drugs, flexible and value-based pricing, market access schemes or risk-sharing models have recently been introduced into some European countries. Additionally, some authors state, that the scarce evidence base, especially for orphan drugs, requires registries [22,23] for long term follow-up. Other suggested solutions to cope with scarce evidence base at the time of approval and the high costs of those niche products include:

Additional studies like phase IV studies or the creation of registries with *all* treated patients to provide more data on its utility, once a drug is on the market. Also, the so called "conditional coverage under additional evidence generation" is increasingly proposed and implemented [24,25]. Since many of the approved orphan drugs (such as Sunitinib, Everolimus, Temsirolimus) are only based on surrogate endpoints (e.g. TTP-Time to Progression, RR- response rate, PFS-progression free survival) a validation using patient-relevant endpoints and the proof of clinical relevancy is still owing [4,26]. The conditional coverage under additional evidence generation therefore seeks to gather data for the final validation.

In addition, it is proposed that if an approved orphan drug consequently develops into a highly profitable blockbuster, a reduction of the exclusivity period should be considered. But a recent EU-commissioned investigation revealed that this might reduce investment incentives substantially [10]. The discussion, if orphan drug pricing may warrant a competition law investigation is ongoing.

Along with the increasing importance of "targeted/personalized medicine", the number of orphan drugs, foremost in oncology, is most likely to increase substantially in the near future. The development of sound and commonly accepted methods (or frameworks) for the assessment of their true risk-benefit profile on the national as well as on the international level is therefore urgently needed.

References

[1] EMA/ European Medicines Agency, *Rare disease (orphan) designations.* http://www.ema.europa.eu/ema/index.jsp?curl=pages%2Fmedicines%2Flanding%2Forphan_search.jsp&murl=menus%2Fmedici-nes%2Fmedicines.jsp&mid=WC0b01ac058001d12b&searchkwByEnter=false&alreadyLoaded=true&status=Positive&status=Negative&startLetter=View+all&keyword=Enter+keywords&searchType=Active+Substance, access May 9, 2011.

[2] EMA/ European Medicines Agency, *Orphan medicines in numbers – the success of ten years of orphan legislation.* http://www.ema.europa.eu/docs/en_GB/document_library/Report/2010/05/WC500090812.pdf 2010. access May 9, 2011.

[3] World Orphan Drug Congress, http://www.terrapinn.com/2011/world-orphan-drug-congress/, access May 9, 2011.

[4] R. Joppi, V. Bertele and S. Garrattini, Orphan drug development is not taking off, *BJCP/ British J Clin Pharmacology* **67**(5) (2009), 494–502.

[5] H.G. Eichler et al., Balancing early market access to new drugs with the need for benefit/risk data: a mounting dilemma, *Nature Reviews Drug Discovery* **7** (2008), 818–826.

[6] R.E. Ferner and D.A. Hughes, The problem of orphan drugs, Editorial, *BMJ* **341**(c6456) (2010).

[7] AMB/ Arzneimittelbrief, *Medikamente für seltene Krankheiten (Orphan drugs).* 42, 2008. 73 (http://www.arzneimittelbrief.de/_anfang/Artikel.aspx?SN=6894, access May 9, 2011.

[8] N. Hawkes and D. Cohen, Drug Regulation: What makes an orphan drug? *BMJ* **341**(c6459) (2010).

[9] F. Godlee, Stop exploiting orphan drugs, *BMJ* **341**(c6587) (2010).

[10] J.C. Roos, H.I. Hyry and T.M. Cox, Orphan drug pricing may warrant a competition law investigation, *BMJ* **341**(c6471) (2010).

[11] C. Wild, Health technology assessment: oncology drugs with orphan designation as an example, *Orphanet J Rare Dis* **5**(Suppl 1) (2010), p. Published online 2010 October 19. doi: 10.1186/1750-1172-5-S1-O17.

[12] A. Denis et al., Policies for Rare Diseases and Orphan Drugs, KCE reports 112C, 2009. www.kce.fgov.be/Download.aspx?ID=2161, access May 9, 2011.

[13] IQWIG/ Institut für Qualität und Wirtschaftlichkeit im Gesundheitswesen, *Welche Evidenz wird für die Erstellung von Leitlinien für seltene Erkrankungen derzeit herangezogen?* Rapid Report, 2011.

https://www.iqwig.de/.../V10-01_Rapid-Report_Evidenz_fuer_Leitlinien_zu_seltenen_Erkrankungeen.pdf, access May 9, 2011.
[14] J. Windeler et al., Zu guter letzt ist alles selten, *Deutsches Ärzteblatt* **107**(42) (2010), 2032–2034.
[15] S. Geiger-Gritsch, *Horizon Scanning in Oncology: Concept Development for the Preparation of a Horizon Scanning System in Austria.* LBI-HTA Report 14, 2008. http://eprints.hta.lbg.ac.at/798/1/HTA_Projektbericht_Nr14.pdf.
[16] A. Nachtnebel, *Azacitidine (Vidaza) for the treatment of myelodysplastic syndromes.* 2009, Ludwig Boltzmann Institut fuer Health Technology Assessment: Vienna.
[17] A. Nachtnebel, *Everolimus (Afinitor) for advanced/metastatic kidney cancer*, 2009, Ludwig Boltzmann Institut fuer Health Technology Assessment: Vienna.
[18] K. Hintringer, Trabectedin (Yondelis) for second-line recurrent platinum-sensitive ovarian cancer, 2010, Ludwig Boltzmann Institut fuer Health Technology Assessment: Vienna.
[19] K. Hintringer, *Plerixafor (Mozobil) for autologous stem cell transplantation in patients with lymphoma and multiple myeloma.* 2010, Ludwig Boltzmann Institut fuer Health Technology Assessment: Vienna.
[20] K. Hintringer, *Nilotinib (Tasigna) for the 1st-line treatment of Philadelphia chromosome positive chronic myeloid leukemia in the chronic phase*, 2011, Ludwig Boltzmann Institut fuer Health Technology Assessment: Vienna.
[21] K. Hintringer, *Dasatinib (Sprycel) for the first-line therapy of patients with newly diagnosed phase philadelphia chromosome positive chronic myeloid leukemia.* 2011, Ludwig Boltzmann Institut fuer Health Technology Assessment: Vienna.
[22] C.B. Forrest et al., The case for a global rare-diseases registry, *Lancet* **26**(377) (2011), 1057–1059.
[23] R. Gliklich and M. Leavy, Patient Registries and Rare Diseases, Applied Clinical Trials, 2011. March.
[24] A. Nachtnebel, Bedingte Erstattung – Erfahrungen aus ausgewählten Ländern, LBI-HTA Report 24, 2009. http://eprints.hta.lbg.ac.at/818/1/HTA-Projektbericht_024.pdf.
[25] C. Carbonneil et al., A common policy framework for evidence generation on promising health technologies, *Int J TAHC* **25**(2) (2009), 56–67.
[26] IQWIG/ Institut für Qualität und Wirtschaftlichkeit im Gesundheitswesen, *Surrogatendpunkte in der Onkologie.* Rapid Report, 2011. https://www.iqwig.de/.../A10-05_Kurzfassung_Rapid_Report_Surrogatendpunkte_in_der_Onkologie.pdf.
[27] U. Schwabe and D. Paffrath, *Arzneiverordnungsreport 2010,* Springer, 2010.

5. Industry perspectives

Pharmaceuticals Policy and Law 13 (2011) 235–241
DOI 10.3233/PPL-2011-0328
IOS Press

Health technology assessment – Plasma product industry view[1]

Charles Waller[a,*] and Robert Perry[b]
[a] *Vice President Europe, PPTA, Belgium*
[b] *Executive Director, IPFA, The Netherlands*

1. Introduction

1.1. Challenges for health care providers

Constraints on health care expenditure is not a new phenomena and most countries with a developed health care sector have experienced progressive year on year increases in delivery costs. The reasons for this are well understood and include increased life expectancy, new high technology interventions and pharmaceuticals, risk reduction measures and general improvements and demands for overall higher quality and access to care. These pre-existing pressures have been amplified by the recent international economic events and by technological advances which offer life extending and enhancing opportunities. Similar pressures apply to developing countries whose populations aspire to benefit from such developments.

1.2. What are HTAs

HTA is a generic term used to describe a range of systems, processes and measurements designed to measure the 'value' of a health care intervention or treatment. HTAs have been defined as 'The systematic evaluation of the properties, effects, and/or other impacts of health care technology'. Evidence used for such assessments includes safety, efficacy, cost, cost effectiveness as well as considerations of ethics, societal values, legal and other implications of new or existing interventions. Therefore to an extent HTAs overlap with well established regulatory processes for medicines and devices (which are primarily focussed on safety, quality and efficacy) but additionally seek to offer health care providers an objective means of establishing cost effectiveness and importantly distribution of finite health care resources

[1] This paper represents the personal views of the authors and not necessarily the views of their associations or members.

*Corresponding author. E-mail: cwaller@pptaglobal.eu.

1389-2827/11/$27.50

across a wide range of differing health care programmes. Typically measurements of value will be expressed as Quality Adjusted Life Years (QALY) facilitating value comparisons between different health programmes.

In one form or another HTAs have existed in many European and other western countries since the late 1970's. However it is only in recent years that such systems have attracted wider attention and application as health care providers and politicians struggle to control escalating health care budgets. Importantly wider political and other local considerations may still play a major role in decision making and overall outcomes.

1.3. Types of plasma products – WHO essential Medicines list – Life saving with clear evidence of efficacy

In any discussion of HTA it is important to emphasise that, for the vast majority of therapeutic products derived from plasma or from modern recombinant technology, their use is life saving and their effectiveness proven and unequivocal. Products for treatment of haemophilia (FVIII, FIX) and immunoglobulin products for treatment of a variety of conditions including immunodeficiency are on the WHO essential medicines list. For patients whose lives depend on the availability of these products there is no alternative treatment and few if any comparator treatment options. In most cases therefore there is a recognition that these products are essential; therefore discussions about these products in the context of HTAs primarily concerns issues of dose, their use in prophylaxis or their clinical value in new indications.

Also albumin products, which were one of the first to be manufactured from human plasma, continue to be regarded as important in the treatment of trauma, resuscitation, and blood loss. Their use and efficacy in newer clinical fields is the subject of (ongoing) research. For example, research into albumin's capacity to bind with toxins and thereby its use in detoxification with related benefits for kidney and liver function and improvement of organ function in patients with sepsis.

2. How do we deal with pharmaceuticals in an HTA process and are there unique characteristics of plasma products which require special consideration?

The plasma products industry has a number of features which make it unique within the wider pharmaceutical/biopharmaceutical industry and in its contribution to health care programmes. The development, over many decades, of safe and effective products primarily for the treatment of rare diseases has transformed the lives of patients who are dependent on these products. Alternative treatments are not available. However these biological products are complex and expensive to manufacture, they are based on blood and plasma donations creating a unique cost structure that rightly requires separate consideration from other modern medicines.

Factors that are unique to plasma derivatives, include the:

- cost of collecting raw material (human plasma) from volunteer donors (whether they are 'unpaid' or 'compensated') which can typically contribute in excess of 50% to the overall cost of product manufacture.
- escalating cost of rigorous regulation, safety measures and precautionary interventions to help ensure product safety which contribute to the overall cost of patient treatment but may deliver increasingly small benefits to either patients or health care providers.
- economics of product manufacture which would be straightforward if the market demand for each plasma-derived product were exactly proportional to its constituent protein's prevalence in human plasma. This however has seldom, if ever, been the case. In practice, disproportionate costs tend to be allocated to those products in greatest demand – currently IVIG.
- absence of any immediate prospect of 'bio-generic' manufacture of plasma products because the quality and safety of such products can be critically affected by minor variations in processing conditions.
- interdependence of: i) each plasma derivative with the others, and ii) the relationship between whole blood collected for transfusion purposes and the production of plasma derived medicinal products.

  i. Plasma derivatives are prepared from the same shared starting material (human plasma), though one derivative will typically drive the overall demand for plasma for fractionation. From the 1960s to the late 1970s it was the need for albumin that determined the quantity of plasma required. This shifted to the need for factor VIII for the treatment of haemophilia A until the mid 1990s when the availability of biosynthetic FVIII reduced the clinical use of plasma derived FVIII in many developed countries and the clinical need for immunoglobulin took over.
  Although one product may determine the total need for plasma, the economic sustainability of manufacturing plasma derivatives requires as many of the therapeutic proteins available from human plasma to be used as possible.
  ii. An important consideration is the interrelationship between blood and blood components for transfusion and plasma derivatives where these share the same donated starting material.
  Virtually all collectors of whole blood separate the various blood components soon after donation. Apart from perhaps 10% of the plasma used directly for therapeutic purposes, the remaining plasma is then transferred to a fractionation organisation. Arrangements for this "transfer" vary widely but most commonly the blood collection organisation receives a payment or it is processed into plasma derivatives for use in the host country. This has the effect of spreading the cost of blood collection over a wider range of products thereby potentially reducing the individual unit costs of the blood components and plasma derivatives needed for various therapeutic purposes.

The plasma product industry is therefore an essential link between donor and patient and even more broadly to transfusion.

It is difficult to see the ways in which comparative effectiveness or health technology assessments can take into account these broader dimensions in a systematic way. Rather, it is proposed that healthcare providers, reimbursement organizations, patients and plasma protein producers work together to ensure that relevant information is fully considered and that unintended consequences are avoided. The interrelationship of all plasma proteins and the interdependence of plasma products with blood for transfusion must be fully taken into account.

Finally it is important to recognise that the industry has duties and obligations to all people who donate the plasma used for fractionation and in particular to maximise the benefit of their donations for patient care.

3. Clinical aspects

There is a strong evidence base for current levels of product use in developed health care systems and best practice guidelines have been developed in many countries to ensure that the use of plasma product therapies are restricted to evidence based indications. However even in these countries there remain serious concerns of under diagnosis in some patient groups, particularly primary immunedeficiencies (PID). The potentially high cost impact of under diagnosis and misdiagnosis of treatable rare diseases on health care budgets (eg arising from the treatment of symptoms rather than the underlying cause) and its wider impact in socio-economic terms (eg limiting the economic productivity of affected patients and their potential societal contribution) are important considerations in any assessment of health care benefits. Identification of these patients must therefore continue to be a priority for health care systems and as a provider of products for such rare diseases, industry should be ready to respond.

Neurological and immunomodulation indications for immunoglobulin are the subject of extensive new research.

Similarly, for coagulation products the research into the role of von Willebrand factor and new work in bleeding disorders in women indicate a growing need. Even in the well accepted indications, the World Federation of Haemophilia[1] constantly reminds us that most people with haemophilia outside of the developed world may receive no treatment whatsoever.

For albumin, new recognition of its therapeutic importance is growing. For example, the potential role of albumin's binding properties is leading an increase in its use.

---

[1] WFH Treatment For All: A vision for improvement http://www.wfh.org/2/docs/About_WFH/Strategic_plan2006.pdf

Finally and despite the advances in developed health care systems it is important to remember that ∼70% of the global population of patients with rare diseases treatable with proven plasma product therapies remain untreated. For these populations HTAs may provide important guidance for countries seeking to improve access to these essential medicines.

The long term global need for plasma for fractionation is neither stable nor predictable. Also the unique nature of the raw material requires relatively long lead times and significant investment to increase its supply.

Thus it is appropriate that when evaluating the clinical and economic aspects of the use of individual plasma derived medicinal products, emerging clinical evidence that may support an increased collection of plasma for fractionation is taken into account as well as the important interrelationships described above.

4. What can the plasma product industry contribute to the process?

We should start by observing that HTAs concerning the use and reimbursement of plasma derived medicinal products are almost non-existent to date. Various reasons, some described in this article, help explain why separate approaches and evaluations for plasma derived medicinal products are needed.

The involvement of industry in HTAs is seen as controversial with some believing that industry involvement will result in a loss of objectivity in assessments and produce an inevitable bias in favour of increased consumption.

An alternative view is that industry is an essential partner in the delivery of care to rare and unique patient groups with an important role beyond that of simply product provider. Indeed consultation with industry is an essential and well recognised part of international regulatory agencies and there is reason to believe that this model and its advantages transfer readily to HTAs. The unique and diverse nature of the industry (both private and not for profit sectors) and its historical involvement with well defined patient groups across many countries and differing health care systems has created a valuable body of knowledge, data and experience which can inform and support HTAs. Clearly such involvement should be transparent. Industry expertise and consultation is already an accepted and valued part of the pharmaceutical regulatory process and there is every reason to believe that this inclusive model can be used to evaluate wider pharmaco-economic issues associated with the use of plasma products.

Examples of specific areas where industry can enhance outcomes from HTAs and health care planning include:

- working with national agencies
- sponsoring and supporting agreed clinical trials
- improving diagnosis rates of rare diseases
- providing data on blood borne infectious disease (HCV, HIV, HBV etc)
- transferring experience from pharmaceutical regulatory activity (which already includes an element of cost benefit analysis)

- contributing to efforts aimed at further integrating regulatory and HTAs – which is already a stated objective of EMA.
- contributing to regulatory decision making to ensure that future/existing regulatory standards are cost effective – important because product costs have a direct and major impact on HTA outcomes.

5. Future prospects and opportunities

Much of the information necessary for conventional pharmaceutical market authorisations and Health Technology Assessments is common to both activities and it is therefore not surprising that Regulators and HTA Agencies are increasingly seeking ways to cooperate and integrate their respective assessment procedure. We can expect to see further integration in coming years. Also there is evidence of increased cooperation and harmonisation between HTA agencies within EU countries and elsewhere.

The future evolution of these activities offers opportunities for both industry and health care providers. These include:

- raising awareness and profile of rare diseases for which there exists highly effective treatment.
- ensuring that available supplies of plasma products (eg IVIG) are used to provide optimum clinical and public health outcomes.
- increasing awareness of the effectiveness of treatment with plasma products and thereby increase availability of products for patients in developing countries.

A key priority for the future should be to increase awareness and diagnosis of rare conditions for which there are proven and highly effective plasma product therapies which would almost certainly produce favourable HTA outcomes.

6. Potential downside risks

As with all measures used to manage health care resources there are potential risks associated with HTAs and in particular their application to plasma product therapies. There are concerns for example that HTAs may not capture the full value and benefit of early interventions with plasma products – for this reason it is vital that patients are represented in HTAs. Also there is the risk of delays in the introduction of new and modified product treatments which, if not recognised, could lead to a barrier to innovation. Finally there are concerns that the involvement of industry in assessments may affect the objectivity of assessments. Open and transparent consultation processes in regulatory developments have mitigated such risks and there is every reason to believe that a similar approach would be successful for HTAs.

7. Conclusions

HTAs have evolved over many years to become an inescapable and important part of the management of health care resources. There is, as yet, little practical experience of their application to plasma protein therapies which have particular and unique characteristics which require an inclusive (patients and industry) approach to their application to ensure appropriate outcomes for both patients and providers.

The outcomes from HTAs may usefully 'read across' countries with comparable and high GDPs and HDI's but may not usefully inform decision making in countries with relatively low HDI's. It may be in the interests of industry, patients and health care providers to support the development of HTA processes in developing countries.

Industry will continue to develop and improve products with measurable patient benefits and favourable HTA outcomes. It is important to recognise that for many of the rare diseases treatable with plasma products most patients worldwide remain undiagnosed and untreated. Therefore industry will continue to support efforts in both developing and developed countries to improve the diagnosis and treatment for patients who unequivocally benefit from plasma protein therapies.

6. HTA perspectives

Pharmaceuticals Policy and Law 13 (2011) 245–251
DOI 10.3233/PPL-2011-0329
IOS Press

Patient involvement in HTA: What added value?

K.M. Facey
Health Economics and HTA, Institute of Health and Wellbeing, University of Glasgow, Glasgow, UK
Tel.: +44 1360 660316/+44 789 414 3931; Fax: +44 1360 660316; E-mail: k.facey@btinternet.com

HTA is an interdisciplinary assessment of evidence and knowledge about the intended and unintended effects of using a health technology. Patients with rare diseases have valuable knowledge about the illness in the real-life setting, but too often their views are seen as anecdotal or biased. So, more needs to be done to elicit patients' perspectives to add value to HTA through effective participation of patients throughout the HTA process and collection of evidence about patients' perspectives through robust qualitative research.

Traditionally HTA has been a broad assessment to move evidence into practice, but in recent years a more limited view of clinical and cost effectiveness has been the focus. For HTAs in rare diseases, this is not enough. Consideration of ethical, organizational and social issues are vital and here patients' perspectives could be particularly valuable to bring a real-life understanding of the potential impact of the health technology.

As countries around the world put more emphasis on creating clear plans to manage rare diseases, we need to ensure that all stakeholders work together to ensure that HTAs are being used flexibly to ensure that there is equity of access to therapies for rare diseases that provide real added value.

Keywords: Patient participation, technology assessment, qualitative research, rare diseases

1. Background

Health Technology Assessment International (HTAi) is a scientific and professional society for all those who produce, use, or encounter HTA. Its mission is to support and promote the development, communication, understanding and use of HTA. It acts as a forum for collaboration amongst all stakeholders; sharing information and expertise amongst members across the world.

The HTAi Interest Group on Patient/Citizen Involvement in HTA focuses on promoting effective patient involvement in HTA. It recognises the need to support patients to be involved in the HTA process and so has developed an HTA glossary for patients [1], which is reproduced in this monograph. The Interest Group has had a paper published outlining best practice [2] in 'patient involvement' in HTA and seeks to share best practice via its website.

The Interest Group believes that 'involvement' is not just about ensuring effective participation of patients in the HTA process, but it's also essential to obtain patients' perspectives in a manner that can be effectively integrated into the largely scientific HTA process (as 'evidence'). These elements of effective participation of patients in the HTA process and contribution of evidence are considered here in the context of HTA for rare disease therapies.

2. Patient participation in the HTA process

Box 1: HTAi Statement on HTA [3]
HTA is the research-based, practice-oriented assessment of relevant available evidence and knowledge on the direct and intended effects of health care technologies, as well as the indirect and unintended consequences. The goal of HTA is to support rational decision making in policy and practice. Generally conducted through interdisciplinary approaches, HTA functions at the interface of evaluation science and policy development. Drawing on a variety of methods and types of knowledge and expertise, HTA is characterized by explicit analytic frameworks and transparency in methods.

2.1. Creating a fair process

HTA is often described as the bridge between science and policy. This analogy is a good one, but the bridge is not a one-size fits all, rigid structure. There is never perfect evidence available to answer a policy question, so the translation of evidence into policy that influences practice requires a deliberative process with value judgments. This is particularly true in the health sector. The evidence available is often limited by the ability to maintain patients in trials long-term and the high cost of research. Meanwhile the policy setting of health systems is complex, with a complex hierarchy of decision makers from the patient, to treating clinician, ward manager and management board of the health provider. Alongside this, there are limited resources, which means that the introduction of a new therapy has a real opportunity cost (that money cannot be spent elsewhere in the system). So in health, the transition from evidence to policy is precarious; perhaps a tight rope walk rather than a stable road bridge.

HTA is actually a complicated deliberative process that balances evidence provided from a range of sources with views and opinions of stakeholders, using value judgments to determine the policy decisions. Many HTA Agencies publish their methods and processes for scientific assessment of evidence, but often their processes of decision-making are less clear.

As Facey et al. [2] explain, effective patient participation in HTA is necessary to create a fair, deliberative process. This requires two-way flow of information throughout the process, not just information-giving or limited consultation on selected components. De Wit et al. [4] recommend that “participation of ‘patient research partners’ should be considered in all phases of the project to provide experiential knowledge, with the aim of improving the relevance, quality and validity of the research process.” Indeed, the HTAi Interest Group promotes the engagement of patients throughout the HTA process, from scoping of the assessment, collection of evidence, evaluation of evidence, consultation and communication. Even before this, patients should be involved in technology development in clinical and post-marketing studies. In all these situations patients can add value.

2.2. *Who are patients?*

When considering patient participation we need to consider what we mean by 'patient'. In general we refer to patients as anyone with personal experience of the medical condition for which the health technology is being used. In our terminology, this includes carers (non professional care-givers). For rare diseases, patient participation seems particularly important, as many rare diseases occur in childhood and for very young children, parents may have more expertise than generalist doctors about the patient's, health, well-being and needs.

The key is that the 'patient' has knowledge about the day-to-day reality of living with the condition, the potential areas where services and outcomes could be improved and can provide valuable insights into the intended and unintended consequences of using a health technology. All seem essential according to the HTAi definition of HTA in Box 1.

2.3. *When should patients be involved?*

For rare diseases, involvement in the scoping of the assessment is particularly important. At this stage the key research questions will be agreed. Researchers want to focus this on available evidence, but that must not be at the cost of avoiding questions that will make a major difference to patients.

Scoping often follows the PICO (population, intervention, comparator, outcome) framework and for rare diseases, patients are likely to add particular value in defining important outcomes. In recent years, there has been greater recognition of the value of patient reported outcomes and good guidance on their development exists [5]. However, it is important to recognize that even if outcomes are reported by patients, they may not necessarily be of importance to patients. This can occur because the perceptions of clinicians and patients about the most important aspect of disease differ. So patients need to advise on patient *important* outcomes [6] that should be studied.

Patients can play an important role in the development of the economic model. In particular, researchers who can elucidate the lack of clarity they have about a treatment pathway could gain valuable knowledge from patients. Patient organizations can also work with their members to determine preferences using standard methodological techniques that lead to utilities [7] and they can be conduits to undertake surveys re costs of care [8].

Many HTA Agencies focus HTA on the assessment of clinical and sometime cost effectiveness. Some HTA Agencies, such as the Danish Centre for HTA (DACEHTA), recognize the value of a wider approach to evidence gathering that seeks to determine the organizational issues associated with the introduction of a new technology into the healthcare system [9]. Any acute health provider runs a complex, dynamic system and DACEHTA use a theoretical organizational model to describe this in terms of structure, functions, staff, technology and stakeholder influences interacting in a context set by organizational culture, financial and legal systems. Patients with rare diseases are often 'experts' on the complex system of care and can elucidate the implications of processes and behaviours on the quality of care that is given and how this may affect technology utilization. So they could provide useful evidence on the organizational aspects.

Some Agencies also undertake explicit analysis of ethical issues and guidance is emerging in this field [10]. As rare diseases are often genetic, HTA should consider not just therapies for rare diseases, but appropriate testing. Networks such as Public Health Genomics (www.phgen.eu) include members from HTA Agencies and some Agencies have started to address the issue of genetics (www.cadth.ca/index.php/en/hta/reports-publications/health-technology-update/ht-update-11/emerging-issues-genetics). However, the focus is often on more common conditions such as diabetes or cancer. For rare diseases, an array of ethical issues may result that affect families and must be considered for new diagnostic therapies. For this a much broader interdisciplinary approach to assessment is needed than is the case for most HTAs.

In terms of assessing evidence, patients can provide clarity about the meaning of an effect and help interpret what the evidence of efficacy (in a controlled study setting) means in terms of effectiveness (in the real world). They can draw out potential benefits and harms that would be of importance to patients. Is it really beneficial – does it allow a return to 'normal daily life' – to work – to family life?

Will we put up with the difficult method of administration and do the harms outweigh the benefits? Such considerations could be important in a finely balanced decision where the value of the technology is questionable. When the technology is clearly high cost and benefit has not been proven, it is unlikely that such input will alter decision making.

For consultation, patient organizations could have a much greater role to play in engaging their members. To optimize this, work needs to be done by HTA Agencies to identify the issues that affect patients and ask them direct questions that can draw on their knowledge and experience.

Communications of HTA findings is a key area where patient organizations could support HTA Agencies, ensuring that easy-to-read summaries of HTA address the issues of concern to patients, make sense and are distributed to those that need that need the information, at the time they need it. This is an area that requires much development in HTA. Lessons can be learned from other initiatives underway in relation to information standards re prescribed medicines in both Europe and the US and from the DECIDE project that will develop methods to communicate clinical practice guidelines to patients (www.decide-collaboration.eu/).

3. Patient evidence

The HEE guide to HTA for patients [11] recognizes that "distress is not enough". Patients who simply lobby for a new technology are often seen as naive (with lack of awareness of the full evidence base) or even worse biased (as many patient organizations are supported by pharmaceutical companies). Hence there is a need to move from emotive views to finding a way that allows robust elicitation patients' perspectives. As happens in the other parts of HTA, a systematic method is needed, using an explicit analytical approach, and findings need to scrutinized.

The optimal approach to achieve such robust evidence relating to patients' perspectives is via qualitative research. A range of qualitative research methods can be used [9], but most popular are surveys, individual interviews and focus groups. Whatever methods are used, the findings should be critically appraised, like any other element of evidence being assessed in an HTA [12].

The interesting thing about qualitative research is that common themes about the experience of living with an illness can emerge quite quickly from interviewing a relatively small number of patients. Hence such methods are applicable to rare diseases.

Of course in very rare diseases, even finding a small number of patients in small countries is a challenge. It is here that the power of web2.0 comes into its own. Blogs and chat rooms can provide interesting perspectives and systematic 'literature' searching techniques are developing to utilize these sources [13]. Several HTA Agencies take submissions of evidence from patient organizations about the burden of disease, experiences of living with the disease, unmet needs and the technology. To obtain such evidence, asking questions of members via a clear survey can be helpful. Alternatively social networking can be used to obtain evidence [14]. This can be achieved by posting specific questions on a social network, summarizing responses and issuing a draft submission for review by the online community. For smaller countries, perspectives could be obtained from neighbouring regions, but care must be taken that the views are transferable and relevant to the health system in question.

4. Discussion

Over the past decade many governments have encouraged a person-centred approach to the delivery of health care. For example in Scotland, the 2005 health plan stipulated that health boards must "develop plans for change *with* people, not *for* them, starting from the patient experience and engaging the public early on to develop solutions rather than have them respond to pre-determined plans conceived by the professionals" [15]. Indeed in Scotland, health boards are judged annually on their mechanisms for public involvement and they must show not only how the public have been involved, but also the difference that their contribution has made.

There have been major developments in the field of HTA in the past decade, but HTA still appears to involve pre-determined plans by professionals, with few opportunities for meaningful patient and public involvement. When evidence is sparse and diseases are complex, as is the case in rare diseases, effective partnerships amongst stakeholders would seem essential to determine the true added value of a new technology and ensure it is provided at the best possible (fairest) price.

Although HTA has developed substantially over the past decade, it has been less obviously patient-centered. It has instead evolved to provide greater transparency of methods of assessment and process. However little has been done to consider how these standard processes can be adapted for new paradigms, such as studying high cost technologies, with high unmet need in rare diseases that have a sparse evidence base. Perhaps one approach is to make use of the emerging trend for early scientific advice that several HTA Agencies are providing to give guidance on study design that takes account of the needs of HTA.

Another important consideration for HTA in rare diseases, is the high proportion of children and young people affected, compared with other diseases. For them evidence may be even more sparse than for a rare disease in adults. Pharmaceutical regulation exists that aims to facilitate the development and accessibility of medicines for children to ensure ethical research and high quality information, whilst recognising that children should not be subject to unnecessary clinical trials [16]. This matter needs to be considered in HTA.

Given the complexity of rare diseases, it would seem essential to take a wider view of HTA as proposed by EUnetHTA [17] in its HTA Core Model, involving nine domains that include organizational, ethical, legal and social aspects. For this, HTA needs to involve a wider range of experts (including patients) and should invest in collection of robust evidence in these fields, in a similar way that investment is made in clinical and cost effectiveness assessments. For these elements, patients' perspectives could be particularly important and qualitative research could influence the value judgments that are required.

The EU has recommended that each Member State establishes and implements plans to combat rare diseases by the end of 2013. Surely as part of this initiative we need to see all stakeholders working together to understand how HTA can be used more flexibly to ensure that it promotes equity of access to therapies for rare diseases that provide real added value.

Acknowledgements

Thanks to all members of the HTAi Interest Group on Patient/Citizen Involvement in HTA who have helped determine and develop best practice for involvement of patients in HTA and worked with passion and commitment to promote that practice internationally.

References

[1] A. Single, Biotext Pty, *HTAi consumer and patient glossary: a beginner's guide to words used in health technology assessment*, Version: 1, 2009. www.htai.org/fileadmin/HTAi_Files/ISG/Patient Involvement/Glossary/HTAiPa tientAndConsumerGlossaryOctober2009_01.pdf (Accessed 18 May 2011).

[2] K. Facey, A. Boivin, J. Gracia et al., Patients' perspectives in HTA: a route to robust evidence and fair deliberation, *Int J Tech Ass in Health Care* **26** (2010), 334–340.

[3] HTAi, *Strategic Plan* 2009–2013. www.htai.org/fileadmin/HTAi_Files/StrategicPlan2009To2013 Materials/HTAi2009To2013Strateg icPlan.pdf (Accessed, 18 May 2011).

[4] M.P.T. de Wit, S.E. Berlo, G.J. Aanerud et al., European League Against Rheumatism recommendations for the inclusion of patient representatives in scientific projects, *Ann Rheum Dis* (2011): doi: 10.1136/ard.2010.135129.

[5] Office of Communications, *Guidance for Industry – Patient Reported Outcomes Measures: Use in Medical Product Development to Support Labelling Claims*, 2009, US Food and Drug Administration.

[6] S. Staniszewska. Patient important outcomes, To be published, 2011.

[7] National Institute for Clinical Excellence, *Guidance on the Use of Beta Interferon and Glatiramer Acetate for the Treatment of Multiple Sclerosis – Technology Appraisal No. 32,* 2002. http://guidance.nice.org.uk/nicemedia/live/11441/32290/32290.pdf (Accessed 21 May 2011).

[8] G. Kobelt, J. Berg, P. Lindgren et al., Costs and quality of life of patients with multiple sclerosis in Europe, *J Neurol Neurosurg Psychiatry* **77** (2006), 918–926.

[9] F.B. Kristensen and H. Sigmund, *Health Technology Assessment Handbook*. Copenhagen: Danish Centre for Health Technology Assessment, National board of health, 2007.

[10] B. Hofmann, Toward a procedure for integrating moral issues in health technology Assessment, *Int J Tech Assess Health Care* **21** (2005), 312–318.

[11] Health Equality Europe, *Understanding Health Technology Assessment*, 2008 www.htai.org/filead min/HTAi_Files/ISG/PatientInvolvement/EffectiveInvolvement/HEEGuideToHTAforPatientsEngli sh.pdf Accessed 18 May 2011.

[12] K. Malterud, Qualitative research: standards, challenges and guidelines, *Lancet* **358** (2001), 483–488.

[13] J. Street, A. Braunack-Mayer, K. Facey et al., Virtual community consultation? Using the literature and weblogs to link community perspectives and health technology assessment, *Health Expect* **11** (2008), 189–200.

[14] D. Wong-Rieger (Consumer Advocare Network), *Using Social Media to Obtain Patient Opinions and Feedback*, HTAi panel presentation (2010).

[15] Scottish Executive Health Department, *Delivering for Health* (2005), Scottish Executive, Crown Copyright. www.scotland.gov.uk/Resource/Doc/76169/0018996.pdf.

[16] European Parliament and European Council, Regulation (EC) No 1901/2006 on medicinal products for paediatric use, *OJEU* **L378** (2006), 1–19.

[17] K. Lampe, M. Mäkelä and M.V. Garrido, The HTA Core Model: A novel method for producing and reporting health technology assessments, *IJTAHC* **24** (2009) S2, 9–20.

7. Glossary

Pharmaceuticals Policy and Law 13 (2011) 255–287
DOI 10.3233/PPL-2011-0330
IOS Press

HTAi consumer and patient glossary

A beginner's guide to words used in health technology assessment

Compiled by Ann Single and Biotext Pty Ltd with contributions from Eleanor Ahern, Tony Culyer, Helena Dahlgren, Karen Facey, Karen MacPherson, Margaret Reid, Karen Ritchie, Tania Stafinski, and Durhane Wong Reiger

Version: 1
October 2009

About this glossary

This glossary explains words that are often used in health technology assessment (HTA) so that they can be more easily understood by anyone, especially patients and consumers. It is hoped that it will inspire clearer communication and support patients and consumers taking part in HTA.

Words that are written in *italics* have their own separate entry. Words that are listed as 'see also' give extra information on the topic.

Patients and organisations are encouraged to use this glossary and provide feedback about its usefulness (please see form at back of glossary).

A

absolute risk reduction	The likelihood that a particular outcome will happen is called the *absolute risk*. The *absolute risk reduction* is the decrease in the likelihood of that outcome due to a treatment or other *intervention*. For example, if a treatment reduces the absolute risk of death from 0.25 (25%) to 0.10 (10%), the *absolute risk reduction* is 0.15 (15%), that is 0.25 minus 0.10 equals 0.15. The estimate of *absolute risk reduction* often comes from clinical trials. The percentage (%) of people taking part that are receiving treatment (treatment group) who experience a specific outcome is compared to the percentage of people taking part but not receiving treatment (*control group*) who experience the same outcome. See *number needed to harm, number needed to treat*

adverse effect A negative or unwanted effect that results from a treatment or *intervention*. Some adverse effects may be predicted as a direct result of the treatment. For example, chemotherapy kills cancer cells, but it may also kill healthy cells such as red blood cells. This leads to the *adverse effect* of anaemia.
Some adverse effects may be the result of incorrect use. For example the wrong dose of the drug may be given or a needle may accidentally puncture an artery.
See *also side effect*

advocate Someone who speaks on behalf of themself or another person.
In health, an *advocate* is usually a person who speaks on behalf of a health care consumer or patient, or a group of *consumers* or *patients*. An example of an *advocate* is a person who is closely involved with *consumers* or *patients* or a consumer support group, and is able to voice any concerns and views of a *consumer* or patient group.

analysis The process of looking for patterns in information to identify cause and effect and/or answer specific questions, such as whether it works and what the risks are. The information is usually collected in research.
There are two types of analyses. *Quantitative* analysis looks for patterns in the form of numbers, such as most frequent choice of treatment option or average rating of pain during treatment. *Qualitative* analysis looks for patterns of meaning, feeling, or beliefs, leading to a finding such as 'most people who support paying more for end-of-life therapy also believe society should give more to those with greater need'.

ARR See absolute risk reduction

B

bias Occurs when a factor influences a research study's outcomes or interpretation of outcomes. There are many types of *bias*. Some are by accident, some are on purpose, some are caused by the research and some are caused by other factors.
Sampling *bias* occurs when the people or entities chosen to represent the entire *population* are not representative. For example, a study that enrols patients on a first-come, first-served basis may be biased towards those who are already receiving better health care.
Publication *bias* occurs because journals are more likely to publish only the results of studies that show a benefit. Studies that show no effect are often not published, even though their findings are just as important.
See *also blinded trial, blinding*

blinding (masking) — A way to prevent the researchers, doctors and patients in a *clinical trial* from knowing which study group each patient is in so they cannot influence the results. The best way to do this is by sorting patients into study groups randomly, for example by pulling numbers out of a hat or assigning them using a random number list made on a computer.
A single-blinded study is one in which patients do not know which study group they are in. A double-blinded study is one in which both patients and the researchers or doctors do not know which study group the patients are in.
One common method of *blinding* is to give patients in the non-treatment or *control group* a similar-appearing fake treatment, also known as a *placebo*. For example, one group might be given an active drug treatment and the other group might be given fake (dummy) pills (a *placebo*).
See *also bias, randomisation*

C

capital costs — The cost of buying and using land, buildings or equipment, and developing the skills to provide a service such as health care.

care giver — See *carer*

carer (care giver) — A person who looks after family, partners or friends in need of help because they are ill, frail or have a disability. The care they provide is unpaid [1].

case-control study — A study to find out the cause(s) of a health *outcome*. This is done by comparing a group of patients who have a disease or condition (cases) with a group of people who do not have the disease or condition (*controls*). The controls should be similar in ways that are not relevant to the causes of the disease or the condition being studied (for example, the same age or living in the same place). This means the researcher can look for those aspects of their lives that differ and may cause the condition.
For example, a group of people with lung cancer might be matched with a group of people the same age without lung cancer. The researcher could compare how long both groups had been exposed to tobacco smoke.

case report — An account of one patient that describes their treatment and the outcome (health condition or disease status).

For example, the report might record the effect of a new type of operation on a particular patient.
See also *case series*

case series (case study) A report on a series of individual patients who have had a specific treatment (such as an operation or a drug). *Case series* do not compare patients with those who have not been given the treatment (*controls*).
See also *case report*

CCA See *cost-consequence analysis*

CCT See *controlled clinical trial*

CEA See *cost-effectiveness analysis*

CEAC See *cost-effectiveness acceptability curve*

CI See *confidence interval*

clinical effectiveness How well a treatment works in the 'real-world' (for example by a doctor with a patient at home), rather than in a carefully *controlled clinical trial*.
A treatment may sometimes be less effective when used outside a trial for many reasons. Patients in the community may be different, may not comply completely with the treatment (because of *side effects* or difficulties in taking the treatment) and may not respond as well as those selected for the *clinical trial*. Treatment recommendations, follow-up and information offered by health care staff may also be different than in the *clinical trial*.
See also *efficacy*

clinically significant A benefit from treatment that relates to an important *outcome*, such as length of life, and is large enough to have practical importance to patients and health professionals. Effects that are identified as *statistically significant* are not always clinically significant, because the effect is small or on an outcome that is unimportant.
For example, a treatment may improve blood flow but for that condition, there is no *evidence* that this leads to an important clinical *outcome*, such as lower risk of blood clots or heart attack.

clinical pathway *Clinical pathway* usually refers to the practices, procedures and treatments that should be used with patients with a particular condition to achieve favourable outcomes. Clinical pathways aim to improve the quality of care.

clinical practice guideline	A document that describes and recommends procedures for the *diagnosis*, treatment and management of a health condition. It is developed to help doctors and patients decide on the best course of action for the patient, taking into account the patient's needs and views. *Clinical practice guidelines* are ideally based on the best available *evidence* for each aspect of health care, as well as agreement between experts and stakeholders.
clinical trial	A study to determine whether a treatment is safe and effective. It is carried out with a *sample* of intended patients, usually after laboratory studies and studies with healthy volunteers have been conducted. The trial is set up to answer one or more questions. For example, does the treatment cause *adverse effects* and, if so, how serious are these? Does the treatment result in desired outcomes for patients, and if so, how much improvement takes place? What is the safest dose to avoid serious *adverse effect*s while still achieving the desired outcomes? See also *experimental study, randomised controlled trial, risk factor*
CMA	See *cost-minimisation analysis*
cohort study	A study with two or more groups of people (called cohorts) with similar characteristics. One group receives a treatment, is exposed to a *risk factor* or has a particular symptom and the other group does not. The study follows the two groups and records what happens. See also *observational study*
comorbidity	Other diseases or conditions that a person has in addition to the disease or condition being treated or studied.
comparative study	A study of two or more subjects of interest such as groups of people who are treated differently for the same condition. For example, the groups might be given different drugs to find out how the different treatments affect the outcome. It can also be a study that looks at the same treatment for different groups (such as different ethnic groups). See also *comparator, clinical trial, randomised controlled trial (RCT)*
comparator	An alternative, or *control*, that researchers use to compare with the test or treatment that is the subject of the study. For example, it may be an alternative test or drug for a condition, or it may be a *placebo* or simply no treatment at all. See also *control*

confidence interval (CI)	There is always some uncertainty in research. This is because a small group of patients (called the *sample*) is studied to predict the effects in the wider *population* who may eventually use the treatment. The confidence interval (CI) shows the amount of uncertainty. It gives a range of results from the study that is likely to include the 'true' value for the *population*. The CI is usually stated as '95% CI', which means that the range of values have a 95 in 100 chance of including the 'true' value. For example, a study may state that 'based on our sample findings, we are 95% certain that the 'true' *population* blood pressure is not higher than 150 and not lower than 110; thus 95% CI is 110 to 150'. See also *confidence limits*
confidence limits	The top and bottom values of a *confidence interval (CI)*. They are the values that define the range of a *confidence interval*. In the *confidence interval* example above, the limits are 150 and 110.
confidentia-lity	The promise not to reveal a patient's information to another person without the patient's consent.
conflict of interest	A situation where researchers or HTA developers have other interests at stake that may influence the results and interpretation of the research; such as financial interests or competition among research institutes or researchers.
confounder	Researchers often look for a relationship between a cause (such as drinking alcohol) and an outcome (such as lung cancer). A *confounder* is a factor that is common to the cause and the outcome of interest (such as smoking while drinking). The *confounder* may hide an actual relationship between cause and outcome or falsely suggest a relationship that does not really exist. For example, researchers used to think that drinking alcohol was related to a higher risk of lung cancer. But, they found that people tend to smoke more when they are drinking alcohol. Smoking is the actual *risk factor* for lung cancer, and is a *confounder* that made it look as if there was a relationship between drinking and lung cancer.
consensus develop-ment	The process of gaining agreement between people, such as a group of experts. Statements or guidelines based on agreement between a group of experts are called consensus guidelines.
consumer	A person who is the ultimate user of the health care resource. A *consumer* may or may not have a specific health issue, condition or disease. A *patient* is someone with a specific health condition. All patients are consumers, but not all consumers are patients.

consumer advocate	See *advocate*
contraindication	A factor (such as high blood pressure or use of another medicine at the same time) that increases the risk of a *side effect* from a treatment. As a result, the treatment will not normally be recommended for people with that *contraindication*.
control	A standard or measure for avoiding *bias* from *confounders* in an experiment. In *clinical trials*, the *control* may be a suitable known treatment (or no treatment), test, *risk factor*, etc. In a *case-control study*, the controls are usually the people without the condition. See also *control group*
control group	The group of people in a study who do not receive the treatment or test being studied. Instead, they may receive the usual treatment or a *placebo*. The results for the *control group* are compared with those of the treatment group to check for any differences. The findings are easier to understand if the *control group* is as similar as possible to the treatment group so that if there is an effect, it is likely to be due to the treatment. See also *control*
controlled clinical trial	A *clinical trial* that includes a *control group* who receive a different treatment from that being tested. For example, the control might be the usual treatment, a *placebo* or no treatment. A *controlled clinical trial* may sort the people taking part into *control* and treatment groups in a random way (based on chance). This is known as a *randomised controlled trial.*
controlled study	A study such as a *cohort study* or *case-control study* in which there is a *control group* matched, for example, by age, sex or where they live. The *control group* does not receive the test or treatment, is not exposed to the *risk factor* or does not have the disease or condition in question. This *control group* is compared with the study group, who do receive the test, treatment or risk factor. See also *control, qualitative research*
conventional treatment	A currently accepted and widely used treatment for a disease or condition.
cost-benefit analysis	This analysis is a method of considering the advantages and disadvantages of alternative health care technologies. The scope of the advantages and disadvantages considered in an analysis depends on the perspective taken. *Cost-benefit analysis* differs from other

forms of economic analysis, like *cost-effectiveness analysis*, mainly in putting monetary values on outcomes.
For example, the costs of an insulin injection may include the costs of the drug, the needle, the nursing time, the monitoring tests and the patient's time. The outcomes (both positive and negative) are also given in terms of money. For example, one outcome may be the savings in potential costs to manage severe diabetes, including kidney failure, circulation and cardiovascular complications, foot problems, and time in hospital. The outcomes might also include the patient's contribution at work, lack of social welfare costs, and increased cost of healthy foods.
The more challenging part of *cost-benefit analysis* is that it assigns money values to outcomes such as better health or improved access. For example, the outcomes might include a monetary value of the expected health gain measured though willingness to pay.
The costs and benefits of a *comparator* treatment are also worked out. For example, the cost of insulin taken by mouth includes the higher cost of the drug, but no cost for needles, and increased cost for more monitoring tests, but no cost for nursing time to make sure patients take it as prescribed. The outcomes of the treatment being compared are expressed as money. For example, insulin taken by mouth saves the cost of being in hospital and long-term organ failure because more patients take it as prescribed. Also included in the outcomes may be the cost of drugs to treat *adverse effects* such as stomach problems.
The difference in costs and the difference in benefits of the two treatments can be directly compared. For example, the total cost of insulin taken by mouth may be more than the total cost of insulin given by needle, but the total savings due to increased benefits may result in total lower costs to the system.

cost-consequence analysis — A type of *analysis* that compares the costs (such as treatment and hospital care) and the consequences (such as *health outcomes*) of a test or treatment with a suitable alternative. Unlike *cost-benefit analysis* or *cost-effectiveness analysis*, it does not attempt to summarise outcomes in a single measure (like the *QALY*) or in money terms. Instead, outcomes are listed in their natural units (some of which may be monetary) and it is left to decision makers to determine the overall balance of advantage and disadvantage.

cost-effectiveness acceptabil- — A method to measure and show as a graph whether a treatment will provide value for money (that is, be 'cost effective') compared with another treatment. It provides more detail about uncertainty in the

ity curve — *cost-effectiveness analysis* than a *confidence interval*. It is based on an *outcome* measure such as a *QALY*.
See *cost-effectiveness analysis*

cost-effectiveness analysis — This analysis compares two or more drugs, devices, tests, or procedures to find out which provides more outcomes for the cost of treatment or which has the lowest cost for a given outcome. This means that the outcomes of all treatments being compared must be measured in the same units.
For example, Drug A for epilepsy results in 90 days without seizure. Drug B costs twice as much, but increases the number of days without seizure to 240. So Drug B gives better outcomes for the money spent as 240 (the outcome) divided by two (the cost) equals 120, which is more than Drug A's 90 days.
Examples of other uniform outcome measures are reduced blood sugar levels, days without cancer symptoms progressing, and years of survival. The more specific an outcome measure the less useful it is in making comparisons between technologies. For example, a measure in terms of cancer symptoms will be less useful in comparing cancer drugs with drugs for multiple sclerosis, so there is a preference for common measures such as life years gained (or *quality-adjusted life-years* gained).
See also *outcome*

cost-minimisation analysis — An analysis that compares the costs of two or more treatments where the treatments have similar effects and only their cost might be different. Costs are, in principle, *opportunity costs* and wherever possible are expressed in money. The aim is to find out which treatment costs the least.

cost-of-illness analysis — An attempt to place a value on the costs, financial and other, of a disease or condition, including *direct costs* (such as the cost of treating it) and *indirect costs* (such as time off work). It does not usually consider the wider costs to society or benefits and outcomes.

cost-of-lost time — The value of the time lost from work due to disease or disability. It is usually based on the average wage/earnings *rate* before tax.

cost-per-QALY analysis — Another name for a *cost-effectiveness analysis* which results in benefits of different treatments or tests being stated as a *quality-adjusted life years*.

cost-utility analysis — A study similar to a *cost-effectiveness analysis*. The costs are measured in units of money and the benefits are stated in a value that

	reflects patient preferences (known as *utilities*), such as a *quality-adjusted life year*. See also *health utilities index*
critical appraisal	A process to find valid and relevant *evidence* or methods in a *systematic review* or *HTA*. *Evidence* is considered using a system of agreed rules to check its quality and decide if it should be included in the *HTA* or not. For example, *evidence* from a particular study may not be included because it is an *uncontrolled study* or uses a different form of treatment from that studied in the *HTA*.
CUA	See cost-utility analysis

D

DALY	See *disability-adjusted life year*
data	Data are the information collected through research. They can include written information, numbers, sounds and pictures. Data are usually stored on computer, so that they can be analysed, interpreted and then communicated to others, for example in reports, graphs or diagrams [2].
Delphi method (or technique)	A technique to obtain agreement from a group, often experts in their field, on a question of interest. For example, in *HTA* it can be used to find out how a technology is being used. The experts answer at least two rounds of written questions about their experiences and current practices in the area of the topic. The goal is to agree on a final group answer (or consensus) on a topic. See also *consensus development*
device	A physical item or artificial body part (called a prosthesis) used to treat a disease or condition or diagnose it. For example, a *device* might be a pacemaker, knee replacement, x-ray or blood pressure kit (but not a drug).
diagnosis	The process of identifying a disease or condition using a test or tests, or by studying the symptoms.
direct costs	The cost to an organisation of providing the test, treatment or procedure. For example, the cost of the drug or the cost of bringing a patient to or from a hospital for treatment. *Direct costs* can be non-medical. See also *indirect costs*

disability-adjusted life year	A measure of the impact of a disease or injury in terms of healthy years lost. For example, the global average burden of disease across all World Health Organization regions in 2004 was estimated as 237 disability-adjusted life years per 1000 *population*, of which about 60% was due to premature death and 40% to non-fatal health outcomes [3].
disease management	The process of managing health and health care and improving *quality of life*, particularly for people with long-term (chronic) conditions. The focus is on trying to reduce the symptoms of a disease and prevent complications, rather than trying to cure it (which may not always be possible).
double blind	See *blinding*
double masked	See *blinding*

E

early warning system	A process for health policy makers and planners that identifies which new tests and treatments are most likely to have the biggest impact on people's health and the cost of providing health care. See also *cost-of-illness analysis*
economic analysis	In *HTA*, an *economic analysis* is an assessment that compares the costs and benefits of using different tests or treatments for the same condition. See also *pharmacoeconomics*
economic evaluation	See *economic analysis*
economic model	A means of estimating the costs and effects of a technology over periods of time or patient groups not covered in a *clinical trial*.
effect size	A measure that shows the magnitude of the *outcome* in one group, such as the study group, compared with that of the *control group*. The effect size is usually tested, using statistics, to find out how likely it is that it is due to chance alone (that is, it is *statistically significant*). For example, if the *absolute risk reduction* is shown to be 5% and it is the outcome of interest, the effect size is 5%. See also *magnitude of effect*
efficacy	The benefit of a test, treatment or procedure gained under ideal conditions, such as in a *controlled clinical trial*.

efficiency	Efficiency refers to either gaining the greatest benefit from a test or treatment using the available resources, or achieving a given benefit in a way that minimises costs. For example, health organisations seek to obtain *efficiency* savings by maintaining the same level of diagnostic service but reducing the number of hospital visits a patient needs to make to for the service.
emerging health technology	A drug, procedure, equipment or item that is not yet commonly used in health care. An example is a drug or piece of equipment that is still being tested in *clinical trials* and is yet to be approved.
epidemi-ology	The study of the diseases that exist in a *population*, their distribution and the factors that aid or prevent their spread. Epidemiology considers the possible *risk factors* for a whole *population* or area, not just the *risk factors* for individual patients.
equity	The principle of treating everyone fairly – that is, not discriminating unjustly against some people. It means recognising that not all people have the same access to opportunities. This may be due to gender, class, religion or age, for example. Equity is different from equality. Equality means treating everyone the same. For example, consider access to care. If all patients are given written information about a test in a country's most common language, the patients are being treated equally. But, it more equitable if each patient is given written information about a test in their language. See also *justice*
equivalence trial	A trial that aims to show that the difference between two tests or treatments is not large enough to matter to patients (that is, it is not *clinically significant*). When this is the case, the tests or treatments are called 'noninferior', and a *cost-minimisation analysis* can be used to find out whether one is cheaper.
ethics	The study of values and customs to understand the principles according to which humans should live. Health ethics describes the principles of good medical practice that determine what is good for individual people and society as a whole. These principles include relationships between patients and doctors, and the use of technology.
evidence	Findings from research and other sources, such as experience, that may serve as a useful basis for decision-making in public health and health care [4].

evidence-based decision making	The process of making decisions about health care informed by the best available *evidence*. See also *evidence-based decision making, evidence-based health care, evidence-based medicine* See also *evidence-based medicine, shared decision making*
evidence-based health care	The process of making decisions about all areas and aspects of health care, such as management and administration, informed by the best available *evidence*.
evidence-based medicine	The use of the current best *evidence* from scientific and medical research to inform the care of individual patients. The *evidence* is used by doctors and other health professionals to inform the health services they provide, and the treatment they offer people who use these services.
exclusion criteria	The features used in *critical appraisal* to decide whether a study is relevant to the assessment. See also *clinical trial, inclusion criteria*
experimental study	A study in which the people taking part are sorted into two or more groups to be given a treatment or test, and then followed up under carefully controlled conditions. Experimental studies, rather than *observational studies*, are the best choice for medical studies because they use *control groups* and minimise *bias*. See also *quantitative research*

F

false negative error (Type II error)	When the statistical *analysis* of a trial detects no differences in outcomes between a treatment group and a *control group*, when in fact a true difference exists in the *population* [5].
false positive error (Type I error)	When the statistical *analysis* of a trial detects a difference in outcomes between a treatment group and a *control group*, when in fact there is no difference in the *population* [5].
focus group	A focus group is a small group of people brought together to talk about a specific topic. Having recorded the focus group, the purpose is to analyse systematically the discussion. It is a good way to find out how people feel or think about an issue, or to come up with possible solutions to problems [2]. Talking in a group results in a different kind of data from that collected in one-to-one interviews.

G

gold standard	In HTA, a *gold standard* is a method, procedure or measure that is widely agreed among the medical profession to be the best available to test for or to treat a disease. New tests or treatments are often compared against the *gold standard.*
gray/grey literature	Information that is not available through traditional peer-reviewed publications, such as scientific journals or books. Examples include conference proceedings, academic report, newsletters, and industry and technical reports. See also *peer review*
guideline	See *clinical practice guideline*

H

health economics	The use of the principles of economics to study health, health policy and the health care system.
health needs assessment	A method of reviewing the top health issues facing a certain group of people. It results in an agreed list of priorities that will improve health care in that area.
health-related quality-of-life measures	A measure of the effects of an illness to see how that illness affects a person's day-to-day life.
health status	The level of health of a person or group of people that is measured either by the person or people themselves and/or by scientific means. The level is usually based on the patients' ability to carry out everyday activities such as dress and feed themselves or freedom from pain. For example, the status may be measured according to whether a person can walk by themselves, walk with a stick, needs a wheelchair or is bedridden.
health technology	Any form of *intervention* to improve health, such as drugs, *devices*, medical equipment and procedures relating to health care and its services, including prevention, *diagnosis* and treatment of a condition.
health technology assessment	The systematic evaluation of the *clinical effectiveness* and/or cost-effectiveness and/or the social and ethical impact of a *health technology* on the lives of patients and the health care system. Its main purpose is to inform health care policy makers.

The process advises whether a *health technology* should be used, and if so, how it is best used and which patients will benefit most from it. Assessments vary, but most look at the health benefits and *risks* of using the technology. They also look at costs and any wider impacts that the technology might have on a *population* or on society.

Health Utilities Index® — A system for measuring *health status*, *health-related quality of life*, and producing *utility* scores [6]. (Source Health Utilities Inc, http://www.healthutilities.com, 4 June 2009).
See also *quality-adjusted life year*

healthy years equivalent — The number of years spent in good health that a patient would see as equal to the actual number of years they spend in ill health.
For example, if someone spent 10 years ill, they may see it as equal to five years spent healthy.
See also *quality-adjusted life year*

HRQoL — See *health related quality-of-life measures*

HTA — See *health technology assessment*

HTAi — Health Technology Assessment international, a non-profit society that supports the growth of HTA community by providing a global forum for the exchange of information, methods and expertise [7].

HUI — See *Health Utilities Index®*

HYE — See *healthy years equivalent*

I

ICER — See *incremental cost-effectiveness ratio*

impact analysis — Evaluation of the affect of an *HTA* on health service organisations or patients [5].

INAHTA — See *International Network of Agencies for Health Technology Assessment*

incidence — The number of new cases of a disease among a certain group of people during a specific period of time [7].

inclusion criteria — A set of conditions that must be met for a person to take part in a *clinical trial*, such as gender, age and type or stage of disease, as well as medical history. It may also be a set of rules to decide if *evidence* is included in a *systematic review* or *HTA*.
See also *exclusion criteria*, *critical appraisal*

incremental cost	The extra cost linked to using one test or treatment over another or the additional cost of increasing the *rate* of activity.
incremental cost-effectiveness ratio	A ratio that shows the extra cost of a more expensive test or treatment, compared with a cheaper treatment or no treatment, divided by the difference in health *outcome*. See also *incremental cost*
indirect costs	The costs that are not directly related to providing the test or treatment. They can be all the goods, services and other resources that are used to provide a test or treatment, or in dealing with side effects or other current or future aspects linked to it. See also *direct costs*
individual patient data	In a *clinical trial*, it refers to the data available for each patient, as opposed to summarised data for a group of patients.
informed choice	A choice made by a person who is judged to be capable of understanding the information available about a test or treatment, as well as its *risks* and benefits. See also *informed consent*
informed consent	The process of a patient or *carer* learning the key facts about a treatment, test or study before deciding whether to agree to it or to take part (such as in a study). Informed consent is an ongoing process throughout the treatment or study to provide information to people, including the potential *risks* and benefits. Informed consent is not a contract, and the person may stop (withdraw consent) at any time. See also *informed choice*
intangible costs	A term often used for a patient's pain and suffering due to disease or illness that cannot be understood as a cost in terms of money.
intention-to-treat analysis	An assessment of the people taking part in a *clinical trial* based on the group they were first put into, regardless of whether they dropped out, followed their treatment to the end of the trial or moved to another treatment. This *analysis* is useful in effectiveness assessments because these changes are similar to the ways patients behave in the 'real world' rather than a *controlled study*.
interim analysis	A report of study data before the study is complete.

International Network of Agencies for Health Technology Assessment	A non-profit organisation that provides a forum for HTA agencies to share information and help stop activities being repeated unnecessarily.
intervention	A procedure, such as treatment with medicine drug, surgery, behaviour change (such as diet or exercise), psychotherapy (such as counselling), early detection (such as screening) or use of patient educational materials.
intervention group	In a *clinical trial*, the group receiving the treatment (*intervention*) in question, as opposed to the *control group*, which receives either no treatment or another treatment.
intervention study	A study that looks at how well a test or treatment (an *intervention*) works. *Randomised controlled trials* are often thought to be the most useful type of *intervention* study to show a difference between *interventions*.
interview	In research, an *interview* is a conversation between two or more people, where a researcher asks questions to obtain information from the person (or people) being interviewed. Interviews can be carried out in person (face-to-face) or over the phone [8]. The *data* from the recorded *interview* would then be systematically analysed.

J

justice	The principle that all people must be treated fairly and equally. See also *equity*

L

levels of evidence	Ranking given to studies based on how well they are designed and conducted. *Clinical trials* with the best levels of *evidence* (that is, trials that have eliminated most *bias*) can then be given the most weight in a review of *evidence*. See also *bias, validity, weighted*
licensing	A marketing authorisation for drugs that assesses quality of production (manufacture), *safety* and *efficacy*.

literature review A summary of the information published in books, journals, etc (the literature) on a topic. A literature review may be a general overview and interpretation of the research, or a more formal review (such as a *systematic review*) of all published studies on a specific topic.

M

magnitude of treatment effect A term that describes the difference between the changes in the study group and *control group* at the end of a *clinical trial* (the *effect size*).

marginal benefit The extra benefit in health *outcome* as a result of adding another test, treatment or resource.

marginal cost The extra cost needed to produce more benefit. The benefit is usually measured as workload or a health *outcome*.

masking See *blinding*

meta-analysis A method often used in *systematic reviews* to combine results from several studies of the same test or treatment to estimate the overall effect of the treatment.
See also *quantitative research*

meta-regression An extension of a *meta-analysis*. A meta-regression looks at the relationship between one or more study characteristics (eg dose, length of treatment) and the *effect size* seen in the studies.

methodology Describes how research is done, including how information is collected and analysed, as well as why a particular method has been chosen [2].

minimisation A way of putting patients into treatment groups in a *controlled clinical trial* that balances the groups in terms of chosen characteristics such as age, sex and severity of disease.

mortality rate The proportion of a *population* that dies within a particular timeframe, for example one year. The *rate* is often given as a certain number per 1000 people.

N

natural unit The actual unit, such as kilogram (for weight), millimetre of mercury (for blood pressure) and score (for pain), that *clinical trial* results are measured in. This is in contrast to units such as *disability-adjusted life years* and *quality-adjusted life years* (which are based on further calculations of the actual measurements).

net benefit The cost of the benefit from a test, treatment or procedure, minus its total costs. For example, if a patient's illness costs $1000 each year in reduced earnings and a treatment costing $100 reduces this by $200 to $800 each year, then the net benefit would be $100 (that is the saving of $200 in earnings minus the cost of treatment of $100).

number needed to harm A measure of how many patients need to have a treatment or be exposed to a *risk factor* for one to have a bad outcome. Ideally this number should be as high as possible because the larger the number the less often bad outcomes occur. It is the opposite *of absolute risk reduction.*
For example, if you give a 100 mg stroke prevention drug to 100 people and two of those people experienced the *adverse effect* of joint pain, the number needed to harm is 50 (that is 100 divided by two equals 50).
See also *number needed to treat*

number needed to treat The number of patients that need to receive a treatment to prevent one additional bad outcome from their medical condition. The smaller the number, the better the *intervention.*
For example, if you give a stroke prevention drug to 20 people before one stroke is prevented, the number needed to treat for that stroke-prevention drug is 20.
See also *number need to harm, absolute risk reduction*

nonrandomised controlled trial A *clinical trial* with a *control group* in which patients are not put in the study group or *control group* by chance (randomisation). Instead, they are sorted by other methods.
For example, they may be put in groups alternately when they arrive for treatment. These methods do not eliminate *bias.*
See also *controlled clinical trial*

O

observational study A study in which a researcher looks at and records exposures (such as tests, treatments or *risk factors*) and observes results (such as the presence of a disease) as they naturally occur. Observational studies can be loosely sorted into two types:

- descriptive studies (such as *case reports* and *case series*) that record how often a disease or condition occurs, so researchers can see the size of a problem
- analytical studies (such as *case-control studies* and *cohort studies*) that look at any links between exposures and results.

In social science, *observational studies* refer to researchers using a system to study people in natural environments to find patterns in their behaviour.

opportunity cost — The increased value of the most highly valued alternative use of a resource. In a fixed budget health care system like that in Canada or the United Kingdom, the true *opportunity cost* of using a resource, such as a nurse's work time, in one way rather than another is the health gain that could have resulted if the resource had been used in the alternative way.

outcome — A test or treatments impact on health or wellbeing.
Some examples of outcomes are the number of patients who fully recover from an illness, the amount of weight that patients lose or the number of hospital admissions. Outcomes are called continuous when the results vary along a continuous scale, such as weight or blood glucose level. They are called binary or dichotomous when the result is either one thing or another, such as improved or not improved, have cancer or no cancer.
Surrogate outcomes are those measured in the short-term that predict longer-term patient-focused outcomes. For example, reducing blood pressure reduces the likelihood of death.
See also *patient-focused outcomes*

outcomes research — Research that seeks to understand the results of particular health care practices and *interventions* in terms of their impact on health and wellbeing – that is *outcomes.*

P

participant — A person who takes part in the research, such as a *clinical trial* in either the *study group* or in the *control group* or a *focus group* or *interview.*
Sometimes, participants are called respondents, patients, subjects, volunteers or *consumers.*

patient — See *consumer*

patient-focused outcome — An *outcome* that is meaningful for patients.
For example, less pain or fewer symptoms may be meaningful to patients, but blood test results may not be related directly to patient outcomes.
See also *health status, intervention*

patient pathway	A plan worked out by a doctor, based on the best *evidence* and patient *preferences*, to manage a disease or condition. The patient pathway specifies each stage of the patient's care, from one point to the next. For example, the pathway starts from before the patient is treated or admitted to hospital, to follow-up after they are treated or home from hospital.
patient representative	See *consumer advocate*
patient selection bias	A type of *bias* where patients are sorted into groups for a *clinical trial* based on factors such as how ill they are, their age or ability to follow their treatment. This may mean that the *control group* is different from the *treatment group*. In this case, any differences the researchers find might be caused by the differences between the groups rather than the test or treatment being studied.
peer review	The critical review of a study by other experts in the area to make sure the study results are accurate and valid. It cannot guarantee that the results of the study will not be flawed (that is, prone to *bias*).
pharmacoeconomics	The *economic evaluation* of the different drugs used to treat a disease or condition, and how much value for money they provide. See also *economic analysis*
phase I, II, III and IV studies	Different phases of *clinical trials* that are run to develop a new test or treatment, such as a drug. Phase I (one) involves using healthy human volunteers to check the *safety* of the test or treatment. In phases II–IV (two to four), patients with the disease that the researchers are interested in are given the treatment and the optimal dose is worked out. Researchers study these patients to see whether it works, how long the effects last and whether there are any *adverse effects*. See also *clinical trial, safety, efficacy*
placebo	A fake procedure or dummy treatment, which looks the same as the real test or treatment, which the people in a *control group* receive. This is to make sure that a study's results show the true effect of the test or treatment.
placebo effect	Any effects in the *control group* that occur because patients expect to get better when they are receiving medical care or due to the extra care given in a *clinical trial*. Researchers must decide whether the effect of the real treatment is greater than the placebo effect. The placebo effect can be measured by treating *control groups* with a *placebo*.

population	A group of people with a common link, such as the same medical condition or living in the same area or sharing the same characteristics. The population for a *clinical trial* is all the people whom the test or treatment is designed to help (such as adults with diabetes, women at high risk of breast cancer). The group taking part in a *clinical trial* need to be typical of the whole population of interest.
preference	A *patient* or *consumer's* personal choice of health care procedures. This choice may be related to lifestyle and other factors that change from one person to another. Doctors need to take account of the patient's preferences when they are developing a treatment plan (*patient pathway*).
prevalence	How common a disease or condition is within a *population* either at a point in time or over a given period of time (it includes new and existing cases). For example, in 2007, the prevalence of diabetes in Scottish NHS boards varied from 3.7% to 4.6%.
prevalence study	A study that looks at how common a disease or condition is in a *population*. See also *prevalence*
primary outcome	The result (s) of most interest to the researchers. A test or treatment can give results for several *outcomes*, but primary outcomes are of greatest importance when assessing the outcome.
primary (research) study	A study that collects data and analyses it. It can refer to either laboratory research or *clinical trials*. See also *secondary study*
probability	The likelihood that an event will occur. In statistics, the probability (or $P-$value) shows the likelihood that a research result could have occurred by chance alone. For example, a $P-$value of 0.05 means there is a five in 100 chance that the effect observed in the trial could have been due to chance. Results with $P-$values of 0.05 or less are usually considered to be a reliable indication of an effect in the wider *population* and are called *statistically significant*.
prognosis	The expected health *outcome* for a person in the future, taking into account their current disease stage, condition or symptoms.
prospective study	A study design where groups of people taking part are followed forward in time. For example, a group of people may be watched to see whether they develop a disease and to see whether this disease

	can be related to exposure to a possible *risk factor*. Prospective studies are slower and sometimes have to be run over many years for diseases that develop slowly. They also cost more to run than *retrospective studies*. Prospective studies give more accurate results because they are less likely to have *bias*.
protocol	A plan that provides the reasons for, and methods of, a study, which must be followed strictly so that the study can be repeated and checked.

Q

QALY	See *quality-adjusted life year*
qualitative research	The act of exploring and understanding people's beliefs, experiences, attitudes or behaviours. It asks questions about how and why. Qualitative researchers use methods like *focus groups* and *interviews* [8]. For example, in a qualitative research study, a researcher might ask people why they want to stop smoking, rather than asking how many people have tried to stop.
quality-adjusted life year	A measure of the state of health of a person or group of people in which the benefits, in terms of length of life, are adjusted to reflect the quality of life. That is, a year of active normal life gained as the result of a treatment is rated higher than a year of living with reduced quality (such as being in extreme pain or being in hospital). It is often measured in terms of the level of a person's ability to perform activities of daily living, their freedom from pain and mental disturbance. The patients, or observers with knowledge in the area, rate these various states by giving them scores.
quality of care	The level of health care provided to a patient or *consumer*. Actions to improve quality of care aim to improve a person's health and meet health care standards.
quality of evidence	How much the results of studies can be relied on to describe a true effect (*validity*). For clinical studies, quality is directly related to the extent to which *bias* has been taken out of the study, which, in turn, depends on how the study was designed and run. See also *critical appraisal*
quality of life	See *health-related quality of life*

quantitative research	Researchers collect *data* in the form of numbers, that is, they measure things or count things. Quantitative research might ask a question like how many people visit their GP each year, or what proportion of children have had a particular vaccine, or whether a new drug lowers blood pressure more than the drugs that are usually used. Quantitative researchers use methods like surveys and clinical trials [8]. See also *experimental study*

R

randomisation	A method of assigning patients to one of several groups in a study by chance, similar to tossing a coin. This method usually uses a computer-generated random number list. See also *random sample*
randomised controlled trial	A study in which the people taking part are assigned by chance (*randomisation*) into groups (such as the *control group* or the study group). The groups are managed in exactly the same way except they are given different treatments, or exposed to a *risk factor* of interest. *Outcomes* are measured at specific time points and any difference in response between the groups is assessed statistically. This method is used to reduce *bias*. See also *controlled clinical trial*
rapid review	A form of HTA done in a shorter time than the usual HTAs produced by the organisation. It may have a narrower focus than the usual HTA, made possible by restricting the specific clinical question(s) asked in the review.
rate	A measure of how often a specific event happens in a given amount of time. For example, during the trial the *side effect rate* was 0.45 (45% of patients experienced a *side effect*).
RCT	See *randomised controlled trial*
recurrent costs	Costs that occur regularly, such as each year, rather than just once, such as staff costs.
reference list	A record of the studies, journals, books, etc, that are used to support a piece of work (such as a study, literature review or article). The reference list is usually found at the end of the publication and provides enough detail for the reader to find and read the pieces of work.

regression analysis	A mathematical or statistical model to work out the effects of an independent *variable* (such as a treatment) on a dependent variable (such as the disease or condition).
relative risk	The *risk* of an unwanted *outcome* in the study group compared with the same outcome in the *control group*, described as a ratio. A relative risk of one indicates no difference in risk between the two groups. A relative risk of less than one means that the test or treatment being studied was effective in reducing the risk of a particular unwanted outcome. For example, if 10% of patients died on the new treatment compared with 15% on the *control* treatment, this is a relative risk of 0.10 divided by 0.15 equals 0.67.
reliability	The ability to repeat a study to get the same result. A reliable study gives a similar result each time the study is repeated with a different *population* or group.
retrospective study	A study that brings together groups of patients with a disease or condition of interest and looks backwards in time. The study examines past exposure to suspected *risk factors* for the disease or condition. Retrospective studies are faster and cheaper than *prospective studies*, but are more likely to have *bias* and *confounding* than *prospective* studies. They are useful if the *outcome* of interest is rare.
risk	The *probability* of an event is the risk of it occurring. Another meaning of risk is the chance that a test or treatment will cause injury or harm. Risks are a product of the effect of a hazard and the level of exposure. See also *risk factor*
risk assessment	A process used to work out what a person's chances are of having a disease or other health condition. Risk assessments usually include four steps: 1. identifying the *risk factor* or hazard (for example, what causes this disease or health condition?) 2. working out how much of the risk factor is dangerous (for example, how high a dose of a toxic chemical is needed to cause injury?) 3. working out how people might be exposed to the risk factor (for example, how and how often, do people come into contact with it?) 4. combining the first three steps to characterise the risk and describe how certain the link is between the risk factor and the *outcome*.

risk factor	Any aspect of a person's lifestyle, environment or pre-existing health condition that may increase their risk of having a specific disease or condition.
risk ratio	See *relative risk*
RR	See *relative risk*

S

safety	The study of *adverse effects* from treatments.
sample size	The number of people needed for a study or *clinical trial*, including the treatment group and the *control group*. In *quantitative research*, the smaller the *effect size* to be detected, the larger the sample size must be. In qualitative research, the sample size may be quite small. The depth in the findings is more important. See also *significant*
secondary research	An academic review of *primary research studies* to gain new insights on a specific topic (such as a *systematic review*).
sensitivity	The *probability* of a positive test result given the patient has the disease being tested for. See also *specificity*
sensitivity analysis	A process that researchers use to check how much the results of a trial would change if the methods for running it were changed or if the *analysis* did or did not include certain data.
serious adverse event	An unwanted effect from a treatment that causes a serious health problem often resulting in the person needing to go to hospital. See also *side effect*
sham procedure	A procedure designed to resemble the real one that is performed on the patient to assess its effectiveness. See also *placebo*
shared decision making	Decisions that are shared by doctor and patient and informed by best *evidence*, not only about risks and benefits but also patient specific characteristics and values [9].
side effect	Any extra effects from a drug, treatment or procedure that are not planned, even when used as instructed. They do not necessarily cause harm. See also *serious adverse event*

significant — Either:

- the difference between results that statistics show are unlikely to have been caused by chance alone (this is called *statistical significance*)
- changes in a person's health condition that make a difference to their overall *quality-of-life* (this is called *clinical significance*).

specificity — The *probability* of a negative test result given the person does not have the disease being tested for.
See also *sensitivity*

staging — Grading how severe a disease is based on well-recognised signs and symptoms and diagnostic tests.

standard treatment — See *conventional treatment*

statistically significant — The *probability* of observing a treatment effect as large as that seen in the sample (such as in *randomised controlled trial*), when there is no treatment effect in the wider *population*, is less than 0.05.
See also *probability*, *significant*

survey — A list of structured questions to collect information on a topic. A *survey* can be done in a variety of quite different ways, such as sent through the mail, delivered face to face or on-line.

systematic overview — See *systematic review*

systematic review — Work that aims to bring together the results of all studies that address a particular research question. They provide a comprehensive and unbiased summary of the research.
For example, one *clinical trial* may not give a clear answer about the effectiveness of a treatment. This may be because the difference between the treatments being tested was very small, or because only a small number of people took part in the trial. So systematic reviews are used to bring the results of a number of similar trials together, to piece together and assess the quality of all the *evidence*. Combining the results from a number of trials (using *meta-analysis*) may give a clearer picture [2].
See also *evidence-based medicine*

T

technology	See *health technology.*
treatment	A procedure administered to improve a health condition.
Type I error	See *false positive error*
Type II error	See *false negative error*

U

uncontrolled study	A study that does not include a *control group*. As a result, these studies tend to be biased and can only be used to help indicate which treatments may be useful. A *case-series* is an example of an uncontrolled study. See also *bias*
utility	A measure of how desirable an *outcome* is, generally expressed as a number between zero and one. For example, a full healthy life would be given a value of one, whereas death is given a value of zero. Utility can also mean a patient's preferred outcome.

V

validity	In a study, *validity* is the degree to which the conclusions that the researchers make can be considered to be 'true', based on how well the study was designed and how well the study matched 'real-life' situations. See also *validity, external; validity, internal*
validity, external	The extent to which the cause-and-effect relationships in a study are true for a wider *population* beyond the study. For example, the external validity of the study may be questioned if the *population* is people in Australia and the study was in Spain, or for old people if the study was in young people. See also *validity*
validity, internal	The extent to which the cause-and-effect relationships in a study are true for the people and conditions of the study. See also *validity*
value	A measure of the desirability or worth of a particular health *outcome* or *intervention*.

variable — A measurement that can vary within a study. Common variables include age, sex and genetic backgrounds of patients.

variance — A measurement of the spread of values for an outcome in a study group. A large variance suggests greater uncertainty in the estimate of the *effect size*, whereas a small variance suggests that a more precise estimate can be obtained.

W

weighted — The influence given to a study or set of data, based on *validity*, size and accuracy or precision.

Background to this glossary

In June 2007, the HTAi Interest Group of Patient and Citizen Involvement in HTA decided to compile an HTAi glossary of terms for HTA for *consumers* .Three members of the sub-group reviewed six existing glossaries to assess their suitability for adoption by HTAi in their entirety or as sources for a compilation. These glossaries were:

1. Australian Safety and Efficacy Register of New *Interventiona*l Procedures – Surgical, date. *Glossary* Adelaide: Australian Safety and Efficacy Register of New *Interventiona*l Procedures – Surgical.
2. P. Richard and M. De Wit, eds, The OMERACT glossary for patient research partners Ottawa: OMERACT, 2004.
3. INAHTA *Health Technology Assessment* (*HTA*) *Glossary*, 2006.
4. The Cochrane Collaboration, May 2005. *Glossary of terms in The Cochrane Collaboration*, Version 4.2.5, The Cochrane Collaboration.
5. National Institute for Health and Clinical Excellence, June 2007. *Interventional* Procedures Programme: Methods guide. London: National Institute for Health and Clinical Excellence
6. National Library of Medicine, Downloaded 9 October 2007. *HTA 101: Glossary*, www.nlm.nih.gov/nichsr/hta101/ta101014.html.

The glossaries were reviewed using the following criteria.

- Readability
  Is the language suitable for a non-specialist? Is there *evidence* that it has been assessed for readability?
- Accuracy
  Is the term defined accurately or could the definition be misleading? Is there evidence that it has been checked for accuracy?

- Usefulness
  Are the terms included of interest to consumers? Is there any evidence of consumer input/involvement?
- Applicability
  Is the term often used by HTAi organisations? Is there general agreement on the term by HTAi organisations?
- Comprehensiveness
  Is the glossary in its entirety suitable for adoption by HTAi?
- Other sources of credibility
  References, descriptions of development processes, etc

More than 1000 terms were reviewed, but few definitions were suitable for a non-specialist audience. Of these terms approximately 200 were considered to be important and applicable for this project and a further 300 terms of potential interest. With funding from the HTAi Board, Biotext Pty Ltd was contracted to prepare a first draft of the glossary. Following a review, this draft was presented to the Interest Group for feedback at HTAi's annual meeting in 2008 and following further work presented again at HTAi's annual meeting in 2009.

Acknowledgements

This work was funded by HTAi under the direction of Ann Single, (Communication and Engagement Adviser, Australia) who undertook all work in a voluntary capacity, with advice from the HTAi Interest Group.

The initial review of glossaries was undertaken by Ann Single, Eleanor Ahern (ASERNIP-S, Australia) and Tania Stafinski, (University of Alberta, Canada).

The first draft was created by Biotext Pty Ltd, Australia.

Subsequent drafts were compiled by Ann Single with input from:

- Eleanor Ahearn, Senior Project Officer – Consumer, Australian Safety and Efficacy Register of New *Interventional* Procedures – Surgical (Australia)
- Professor Tony Culyer, Ontario Chair of Health Policy and System Design, University of Toronto (Canada), Professor of Economics, University of York (UK)
- Helena Dahlgren, Deputy Director/Project Director, Swedish Council on Technology Assessment in Health Care SBU (Sweden)
- Dr Karen Facey, Evidence Based Health Policy Consultant (Scotland, UK), Chair, HTAi Interest Group of Patient and Citizen Involvement in HTA
- Karen MacPherson, Health Services Researcher, NHS Quality Improvement Scotland (UK)
- Professor Margaret Reid, FFPH Professor of Women's Health Public Health and Health Policy University of Glasgow (Scotland, UK)

- Dr Karen Ritchie, Lead Health Service Research, NHS Quality Improvement Scotland (UK)
- Tania Stafinski, Research Program Coordinator, Department of Public Health Sciences, University of Alberta (Canada).
- Dr Durhane Wong-Rieger, President and CEO, Anemia Institute for Research and Education Institute for Optimizing Health Outcomes (Canada)

And expert advice from:

- Antoine Boivin MD, MSc CCFP, Scientific Institute for Quality of Healthcare (The Netherlands)
- Javier Gracia MD, MPH, Researcher, Health Technology Assessment Unit (UETS), Agencia Laín Entralgo, Ministry of Health of Madrid, (Spain)
- Dr Birthe Jorgensen, Director, Medical Advisory Secretariat, Ministry of Health and Long-Term Care, Ontario (Canada)

Please tell us what you think of this glossary

By filling in this form and faxing it to: 0131 225 5558 (if in the UK) or +44 131 225 5558 (if not in the UK)

Please circle the answer that best matches your view.

1. The glossary is useful.
   Strongly agree Agree Not sure Disagree Strongly disagree

2. The glossary helped me to understand health technology assessment.
   Strongly agree Agree Not sure Disagree Strongly disagree
3. The glossary is easy to understand.
   Strongly agree Agree Not sure Disagree Strongly disagree
4. Were there terms you found hard to understand? Yes □ No □
   If yes, which terms were they?
   ______________________ ______________________
   ______________________ ______________________
   ______________________ ______________________
   ______________________ ______________________

5. Are there any terms you would like to see added to the glossary?
   ______________________ ______________________
   ______________________ ______________________
   ______________________ ______________________
   ______________________ ______________________

6. The glossary was made for people to look up terms and find out what they mean. Is this how you used it? Yes □ No □
   If not, how did you use it?
   ____

____

____

7. The glossary would be better if . . .

   ____

   ____

   ____

8. Any other comments?

   ____

   ____

   ____

9. Can you tell us a bit more about yourself?
   Age group:
   Under 20 20–29 30–39 40–49 50–59 60–69 70 +
   First language: _______________________________
   How would you describe yourself (please circle):
   Patient Health professional Researcher
   Consumer Other _______________________________
10. If you would like to know when the glossary is updated, please provide your email address: _______________________________
    □ Please tick this box if you would to know more about the HTAi Interest Group for Patient and Citizen Involvement

Feedback form for organisations trialling the glossary

By filling in this form and faxing it to: 0131 225 5558 (if in the UK) or +44 131 225 5558 (if not in the UK)

Please circle the answer that best matches your view.

1. The glossary is useful for members of our organisation.
   Strongly agree Agree Not sure Disagree Strongly disagree
2. The glossary definitions are accurate.
   Strongly agree Agree Not sure Disagree Strongly disagree
3. The language in the glossary is appropriate for members of our organisation.
   Strongly agree Agree Not sure Disagree Strongly disagree
4. Were there terms you found hard to understand? Yes □ No □
   If yes, which terms were they?

   ____________________ ____________________

   ____________________ ____________________

   ____________________ ____________________

   ____________________ ____________________

5. Are there any terms you would like to see added to the glossary?

   ____________________ ____________________

______________________ ______________________
______________________ ______________________
______________________ ______________________

6. How did your organisation use the glossary?
____
____

7. The glossary would be better if . . .
____
____
____

8. Any other comments?
____
____
____

9. What sort of organisation do you represent?
____

10. If you would like to know when the glossary is updated, please provide your email address: ______________________

    □ Please tick this box if you would to know more about the HTAi Interest Group for Patient and Citizen Involvement

    Optional

    Name: E-mail: ______________________

References

[1] NHS Quality Improvement Scotland Glossary, www.nhshealthquality.org/nhsqis/723.html (downloaded 3 June 2009).

[2] S. Adapted from Buckland et al., 2007. *Public Information Pack. How to get actively involved in NHS, public health and social care research*. London: INVOLVE.

[3] World Health Organisation, 2004. *The Global Burden of Disease: 2004 Update* World Health Organisation

[4] Adapted from: European Advisory Committee on Health Research (EACHR). Considerations in defining evidence for public health, *International Journal of Technology Assessment in Health Care* **19**(3) (2003), 559–573.

[5] International Network of Agencies for Health Technology Assessment, 2006. Health Technology Assessment (HTA) Glossary. Stockholm: International Network of Agencies for Health Technology Assessment.

[6] Health Utilities Inc., www.healthutilities.com (downloaded 4 June 2009).

[7] I. Bradbury, E. Bonell, J. Boynton, E. Cummins, K. Facey, K. Iqbal, G. Laking, C. McDonald, T. Parpia, P. Sharp, A. Single and A. Walker, Positron emission tomography (PET) imaging in cancer management. Health Technology Assessment Report 2. Glasgow: Health Technology Board for Scotland, 2002.

[8] S. Buckland et al., Public Information Pack. How to get actively involved in NHS, public health and social care research. INVOLVE, 2007.

[9] A. Towle and W. Godolphin, Framework for teaching and learning informed shared decision making, *BMJ* **319** (1999), 766–771.

Appendices

Pharmaceuticals Policy and Law 13 (2011) 291–298
DOI 10.3233/PPL-2011-0331
IOS Press

Council Directive 89/105/EEC of 21 December 1988 relating to the transparency of measures regulating the prices of medicinal products for human use and their inclusion in the scope of national health insurance systems

Official Journal L 040 , 11/02/1989 P. 0008 – 0011
Finnish special edition: Chapter 15 Volume 9 P. 0045
Swedish special edition: Chapter 15 Volume 9 P. 0045

THE COUNCIL OF THE EUROPEAN COMMUNITIES,

Having regard to the Treaty establishing the European Economic Community, and in particular Article 100a thereof,

Having regard to the proposal from the Commission [1],

In cooperation with the European Parliament [2],

Having regard to the opinion of the Economic and Social Committee [3],

Whereas marketing authorizations for proprietary medicinal products issued pursuant to Council Directive 6S/65/EEC of 26 January 1965 on the approximation of provisions laid down by law, regulation or administrative action relating to proprietary medicinal products [4], as last amended by Directive 87/21/EEC [5], may be refused only for reasons relating to the quality, safety or efficacy of the proprietary medicinal productsconcerned:

Whereas Member States have adopted measures of an economic nature on the marketing ofmedicinal productsin order to control public health expenditure on such products; whereas such measures include direct and indirect controls on the prices of medicinal products as a consequence of the inadequacy or absence of competition in the medicinal products market and limitations on the range of products covered by national health insurance systems;

Whereas the primary objective of such measures is the promotion of public health by ensuring the availability of adequate supplies of medicinal products at a reasonable cost; whereas, however, such measures should also be intended to promote efficiency in the production of medicinal products and to encourage research and development into new medicinal products, on which the maintenance of a high level of public health within the Community ultimately depends;

Whereas disparities in such measures may hinder or distort intra-Community trade in medicinal products and thereby directly affect the functioning of the common market in medicinal products;

Whereas the objective of this Directive is to obtain an overall view of national pricing arrangements, including the manner in which they operate in individual cases and all the criteria on which they are based, and to provide public access to them for all those involved in the market in medicinal products in the Member States; whereas this information should be public;

Whereas, as a first step towards the removal of these disparites, it is urgently necessary to lay down a series of requirements intended to ensure that all concerned can verify that the national measures do not constitute quantatative restrictions on imports or exports or measures having equivalent effect thereto; whereas, however, these requirements do not effect the policies of those Member States which rely primarily upon free competition to determine the price of medicinal products; whereas these requirements also do not affect national policies on price setting and on the determination of social security schemes, except as far as it is necessary to attain transparency within the meaning of this Directive;

Whereas the further harmonization of such measures must take place progressively,

HAS ADOPTED THIS DIRECTIVE:

Article 1

1. Member States shall ensure that any national measure, whether laid down by law, regulation or administrative action, to control the prices of medicinal products for human use or to restrict the range of medicinal products covered by their national health insurance systems complies with the requirements of this Directive.
2. The definition of 'medicinal products' laid down in Article 1 of Directive 65/65/EEC shall apply to this Directive.
3. Nothing in this Directive shall permit the marketing of a proprietary medicinal product in respect of which the authorization provided for in Article 3 of Directive 65/65/EEC has not been issued.

Article 2

The following provisions shall apply if the marketing of a medicinal product is permitted only after the competent authorities of the Member State concerned have approved the price of the product:

1. Member States shall ensure that a decision on the price which may be charged for the medicinal product concerned is adopted and communicated to the applicant within 90 days of the receipt of an application submitted, in accordance with the requirements laid down in the Member State concerned, by the holder of a marketing authorization. The applicant shall furnish the competent authorities with adequate information. If the information supporting the application

is inadequate, the competent authorities shall forthwith notify the applicant of what detailed additional information is required and take their final decision within 90 days of receipt of this additional information. In the absence of such a decision within the abovementioned period or periods, the applicant shall be entitled to market the product at the price proposed

2. Should the competent authorities decide not to permit the marketing of the medicinal product concerned at the price proposed by the applicant, the decision shall contain a statement of reasons based on objective and verifiable criteria. In addition, the applicant shall be informed of the remedies available to him under the laws in force and the time limits allowed for applying for such remedies.
3. At least once a year, the competent authorities shall publish in an appropriate publication, and communicate to the Commission, a list of the medicinal products the price of which has been fixed during the relevant period, together with the prices which may be charged for such products.

Article 3

Without prejudice to Article 4, the following provisions shall apply if an increase in the price of a medicinal product is permitted only after prior approval has been obtained from the competent authorities:

1. Member States shall ensure that a decision is adopted on an application submitted, in accordance with the requirements laid down in the Member State concerned, by the holder of a marketing authorization to increase the price of a medicinal product and communicated to the applicant within 90 days of its receipt. The applicant shall furnish the competent authorities with adequate information including details of those events intervening since the price of the medicinal product was last determined which in his opinion justify the price increase requested. If the information supporting the application is inadequate, the competent authorities shall forthwith notify the applicant of what detailed additional information is required and take their final decision within 90 days of receipt of this additional information.
   In case of an exceptional number of applications, the period may be extended once only for a further 60 days. The applicant shall be notified of such extension before the expiry of the period.
   In the absence of such a decision within the abovementioned period or periods, the applicant shall be etitled to apply in full the price increase requested
2. Should the competent authorities decide not to permit the whole or part of the price increase requested, the decision shall contain a statement of reasons based on objective and verifiable criteria and the applicant shall be informed of the remedies available to him under the laws in force and the time limits allowed for applying for such remedies.

3. At least once a year, the competent authorities shall publish in an appropriate publication and communicate to the Commission, a list of the medicinal products for which price increases have been granted during the relevant period, together with the new price which may be charged for such products.

Article 4

1. In the event of a price freeze imposed on all medicinal products or on certain categories of medicinal products by the competent authorities of a Member State, that Member State shall carry out a review, at least once a year, to ascertain whether the macro-economic conditions justify that the freeze be continued unchanged. Within 90 days of the start of this review, the competent authorities shall announce what increases or decreases in prices are being made, if any.
2. In exceptional cases, a person who is the holder of a marketing authorization for a medicinal product may apply for a derogation from a price freeze if this is justified by particular reasons. The application shall contain an adequate statement of these reasons. Member States shall ensure that a reasoned decision on any such application is adopted and communicated to the applicant within 90 days. If the information supporting the application is inadequate, the competent authorities shall forthwith notify the applicant of what detailed additional information is required and take their final decision within 90 days of receipt of this additional information. Should the derogation be granted, the competent authorities shall forthwith publish an announcement of the price increase allowed.

Should there be an exceptional number of applications, the period may be extended once only for a further 60 days. The applicant shall be notified of such extension before the expiry of the initial period.

Article 5

Where a Member State adopts a system of direct or indirect controls on the profitability of persons responsible for placing medicinal products on the market, the Member State concerned shall publish the following information in an appropriate publication and communicate it to the Commission:

(a) the method or methods used in the Member State concerned to define profitability: return on sales and/or return on capital;
(b) the range of target profit currently permitted to persons responsible for placing medicinal products on the market in the Member State concerned;
(c) the criteria according to which target rates of profit are accorded to an individual responsible for placing medicinal products on the market, together with the criteria according to which they will be allowed to retain profits above their given targets in the Member State concerned;

(d) the maximum percentage profit which any person responsible for placing medicinal products von the market is allowed to retain above his target in the Member State concerned

This information shall be updated once a year or when significant changes are made.

Where, in addition to operating a system of direct or indirect controls on profits, a Member State operates a system of controls on the prices of certain types of medicinal products which are excluded from the scope of the profit control scheme, Articles 2, 3 and 4 shall, where relevant, apply to such price controls. However, the said Articles shall not apply where the normal operation of a system of direct or indirect controls on profits results exceptionally in a price being fixed for an individual medicinal product.

Article 6

The following provisions shall apply if a medicinal product is covered by the national health insurance system only after the competent authorities have decided to include the medicinal product concerned in a positive list of medicinal products covered by the national health insurance system.

1. Member States shall ensure that a decision on an application submitted, in accordance with the requirements laid down in the Member State concerned, by the holder of a marketing authorization to include a medicinal product in the list of medicinal products covered by the health insurance systems is adopted and communicated to the applicant within 90 days of its receipt. Where an application under this Article may be made before the competent authorities have agreed the price to be charged for the product pursuant to Article 2, or where a decision on the price of a medicinal product and a decision on its inclusion within the list of products covered by the health insurance system are taken after a single administrative procedure, the time limit shall be extended for a further 90 days. The applicant shall furnish the competent authorities with adequate information. If the information supporting the application is inadequate, the time limit shall he suspended and the competent authorities shall forthwith notify the applicant of what detailed additional information is required.
   Where a Member State does not permit an application to be made under this Article before the competent authorities have agreed the price to be charged for the product pursuant to Article 2, the Member State concerned shall ensure that the overall period of time taken by the two procedures does not exceed 180 days. This time limit may be extended in accordance with Article 2 or suspended in accordance with the provisions of the preceding subparagraph.
2. Any decision not to include a medicinal product in the list of products covered by the health insurance system shall contain a statement of reasons based upon

objective and verifiable criteria, including, if appropriate, any expert opinions or recommendations on which the decision is based. In addition, the applicant shall be informed of the remedies available to him under the laws in force and of the time limits allowed for applying for such remedies.

3. Before the date referred to in Article 11 [1], Member States shall publish in an appropriate publication and communicate to the Commission the criteria which are to be taken into account by the competent authorities in deciding whether or not to include medicinal products on the lists.
4. Within one year of the date referred to in in Article 11 [1], Member States shall publish in an appropriate publication and communicate to the Commission a complete list of the products covered by their healeh insurance system, together with their prices fixed by the national competent authorities. This information shall be updated at least once every year.
5. Any decision to exclude a product from the list of products covered by the health insurance system shall contain a statement of reasons based on objective and verifiable criteria. Such decisions, including, if appropriate, any expert opinions or recommendations on which the decisions are based, shall be communicated to the person responsible, who shall be informed of the remedies available to him under the laws in force and the time limits allowed for applying for such remedies.
6. Any decision to exclude a category of medicinal products from the list of products covered by the health insurance system shall contain a statement of reasons based on objective and verifiable criteria and be published in an appropriate publication.

Article 7

The following provisions shall apply if the competent authorities of a Member State are empowered to adopt.

decisions to exclude individual or categories of medicinal products from the coverage of its national health insurance system (negative lists).

1. Any decision to exclude a category of medicinal products from the coverage of the national health insurance system shall contain a statement of reasons based upon objective and verifiable criteria and be published in an appropriate publication.
2. Before the date referred to in Article 11 [1], Member States shall publish in an appropriate publication and communicate to the Commission the criteria which are to be taken into account by the competent authorities in deciding whether or not to exclude an individual medicinal product from the coverage of the national health insurance system.
3. Any decision to exclude an individual medicinal product from the coverage of the national health insurance system shall contain a statement of reasons based

on objective and verifiable criteria. Such decisions, including, if appropriate, any expert opinions or recommendations on which the decisions are based, shall be communicated to the person responsible, who shall be informed of the remedies available to him under the laws in force and the time limits allowed for applying for such remedies.

4. Within one year of the date referred to in Article 11 [1], the competent authorities shall publish in an appropriate publication and communicate to the Commission a list of the individual medicinal products which have been excluded from the scope of its health insurance system. This information shall be updated at least every six months.

Article 8

1. Before the date referred to in Article 11 [1], Member States shall communicate to the Commission any criteria concerning the therapeutic classification of medicinal products which are used by the competent authorities for the purposes of the national social security system.
2. Before the date referred to in Article 11 [1], Member States shall communicate to the Commission any criteria which are used by the competent authorities in verifying the fairness and transparency of the prices charged for transfers within a group of companies of active principles or intermediate products used in the manufacture of medicinal products or finished medicinal products.

Article 9

1. In the light of experience, the Commission shall, not later than two years after the date referred to in Article 11 [1], submit to the Council a proposal containing appropriate measures leading towards the abolition of any remaining barriers to, or distortions of, the free movement of proprietary medicinal products, so as to bring this sector closer into line within the normal conditions of the internal market.
2. The Council shall decide on the Commission proposal not later than one year after its submission.

Article 10

1. A Committee called the 'Consultative Committee for the implementation of Directive 89/105/EEC relating to the transparency of measures regulating the pricing of medicinal products for human use and their inclusion in the scope of national health insurance systems' shall be set up and attached to the Commission.
2. The tasks of the committee shall be to examine any question relating to the application of this Directive which is brought up by the Commission or at the request of a Member State.

3. The committee shall consist of one representative from each Member State. There shall be one deputy for each representative. This deputy shall be entitled to participate in meetings of the committee.
4. A representative of the Commission shall chair the committee.
5. The committee shall adopt its rules of procedure.

Article 11

1. Member States shall bring into force the laws, regulations and administrative provisions necessary to comply with this Directive by 31 December 1989 at the latest. They shall forthwith inform the Commission thereof.
2. Before the date referred to in paragraph 1, Member States shall communicate to the Commission the texts of any laws, regulations or administrative provisions relating to the pricing of medicinal products, the profitability of manufacturers of medicinal products and the coverage of medicinal products by the national health insurance system Amendments and modifications to these laws, regulations or administrative provisions shall be communicated to the Commission forthwith.

Article 12

This Directive is addressed to the Member States
Done at Brussels, 21 December 1989
For the Council
The President

References

[1] OJ, N°C 17, 23. 1. 1987, p. 6 and OJ N° 129, 18. 5. 1988, p. 14.
[2] OJ N°C 94, 11. 4. 1988, p. 62 and OJ N°C 326, 19. 12. 1988.
[3] OJ N°C 319, 30. 11. 1987, p. 47.
[4] OJ N° 22, 9. 2. 1965, p. 369/65.
[5] OJ N° L 1S, 17. 1. 1987, p. 36.

Pharmaceuticals Policy and Law 13 (2011) 299–300
DOI 10.3233/PPL-2011-0334
IOS Press

Public Health. Title XIV. Article 168. (ex Article 152 TEC). Treaty on the Functioning of the European Union[1]

1. A high level of human health protection shall be ensured in the definition and implementation of all Union policies and activities.
   Union action, which shall complement national policies, shall be directed towards improving public health, preventing physical and mental illness and diseases, and obviating sources of danger to physical and mental health. Such action shall cover the fight against the major health scourges, by promoting research into their causes, their transmission and their prevention, as well as health information and education, and monitoring, early warning of and combating serious cross-border threats to health.
   The Union shall complement the Member States' action in reducing drugs-related health damage, including information and prevention.
2. The Union shall encourage cooperation between the Member States in the areas referred to in this Article and, if necessary, lend support to their action. It shall in particular encourage cooperation between the Member States to improve the complementarity of their health services in cross-border areas.
   Member States shall, in liaison with the Commission, coordinate among themselves their policies and programmes in the areas referred to in paragraph 1. The Commission may, in close contact with the Member States, take any useful initiative to promote such coordination, in particular initiatives aiming at the establishment of guidelines and indicators, the organisation of exchange of best practice, and the preparation of the necessary elements for periodic monitoring and evaluation.
   The European Parliament shall be kept fully informed.
3. The Union and the Member States shall foster cooperation with third countries and the competent international organisations in the sphere of public health.
4. By way of derogation from Article 2(5) and Article 6(a) and in accordance with Article 4(2)(k) the European Parliament and the Council, acting in accordance with the ordinary legislative procedure and after consulting the Economic and Social Committee and the Committee of the
   Regions, shall contribute to the achievement of the objectives referred to in this Article through adopting in order to meet common safety concerns:
   (a) measures setting high standards of quality and safety of organs and substances of human origin, blood and blood derivatives; these measures shall not prevent any Member State from maintaining or introducing more stringent protective measures;

(b) measures in the veterinary and phytosanitary fields which have as their direct objective the protection of public health;
(c) measures setting high standards of quality and safety for medicinal products and devices for medical use.

5. The European Parliament and the Council, acting in accordance with the ordinary legislative procedure and after consulting the Economic and Social Committee and the Committee of the
Regions, may also adopt incentive measures designed to protect and improve human health and in particular to combat the major cross-border health scourges, measures concerning monitoring, early warning of and combating serious cross-border threats to health, and measures which have as their direct objective the protection of public health regarding tobacco and the abuse of alcohol, excluding any harmonisation of the laws and regulations of the Member States.
6. The Council, on a proposal from the Commission, may also adopt recommendations for the purposes set out in this Article.
7. Union action shall respect the responsibilities of the Member States for the definition of their health policy and for the organisation and delivery of health services and medical care. The responsibilities of the Member States shall include the management of health services and medical care and the allocation of the resources assigned to them. The measures referred to in paragraph 4(a) shall not affect national provisions on the donation or medical use of organs and blood.

30.3.2010 EN Official Journal of the European Union C 83/123
Consolidated version of the Treaty on the Functioning of the European Union
123

Pharmaceuticals Policy and Law 13 (2011) 301–310
DOI 10.3233/PPL-2011-0332
IOS Press

Council Directive 2000/43/EC of 29 June 2000 implementing the principle of equal treatment between persons irrespective of racial or ethnic origin

Official Journal L 180, 19/07/2000 P. 0022 – 0026

THE COUNCIL OF THE EUROPEAN UNION,

Having regard to the Treaty establishing the European Community and in particular Article 13 thereof,
Having regard to the proposal from the Commission(1),
Having regard to the opinion of the European Parliament(2),
Having regard to the opinion of the Economic and Social Committee(3),
Having regard to the opinion of the Committee of the Regions(4),
Whereas:

(1) The Treaty on European Union marks a new stage in the process of creating an ever closer union among the peoples of Europe.
(2) In accordance with Article 6 of the Treaty on European Union, the European Union is founded on the principles of liberty, democracy, respect for human rights and fundamental freedoms, and the rule of law, principles which are common to the Member States, and should respect fundamental rights as guaranteed by the European Convention for the protection of Human Rights and Fundamental Freedoms and as they result from the constitutional traditions common to the Member States, as general principles of Community Law.
(3) The right to equality before the law and protection against discrimination for all persons constitutes a universal right recognised by the Universal Declaration of Human Rights, the United Nations Convention on the Elimination of all forms of Discrimination Against Women, the International Convention on the Elimination of all forms of Racial Discrimination and the United Nations Covenants on Civil and Political Rights and on Economic, Social and Cultural Rights and by the European Convention for the Protection of Human Rights and Fundamental Freedoms, to which all Member States are signatories.
(4) It is important to respect such fundamental rights and freedoms, including the right to freedom of association. It is also important, in the context of the access to and provision of goods and services, to respect the protection of private and family life and transactions carried out in this context.
(5) The European Parliament has adopted a number of Resolutions on the fight against racism in the European Union.

(6) The European Union rejects theories which attempt to determine the existence of separate human races. The use of the term "racial origin" in this Directive does not imply an acceptance of such theories.

(7) The European Council in Tampere, on 15 and 16 October 1999, invited the Commission to come forward as soon as possible with proposals implementing Article 13 of the EC Treaty as regards the fight against racism and xenophobia.

(8) The Employment Guidelines 2000 agreed by the European Council in Helsinki, on 10 and 11 December 1999, stress the need to foster conditions for a socially inclusive labour market by formulating a coherent set of policies aimed at combating discrimination against groups such as ethnic minorities.

(9) Discrimination based on racial or ethnic origin may undermine the achievement of the objectives of the EC Treaty, in particular the attainment of a high level of employment and of social protection, the raising of the standard of living and quality of life, economic and social cohesion and solidarity. It may also undermine the objective of developing the European Union as an area of freedom, security and justice.

(10) The Commission presented a communication on racism, xenophobia and anti-Semitism in December 1995.

(11) The Council adopted on 15 July 1996 Joint Action (96/443/JHA) concerning action to combat racism and xenophobia(5) under which the Member States undertake to ensure effective judicial cooperation in respect of offences based on racist or xenophobic behaviour.

(12) To ensure the development of democratic and tolerant societies which allow the participation of all persons irrespective of racial or ethnic origin, specific action in the field of discrimination based on racial or ethnic origin should go beyond access to employed and self-employed activities and cover areas such as education, social protection including social security and healthcare, social advantages and access to and supply of goods and services.

(13) To this end, any direct or indirect discrimination based on racial or ethnic origin as regards the areas covered by this Directive should be prohibited throughout the Community. This prohibition of discrimination should also apply to nationals of third countries, but does not cover differences of treatment based on nationality and is without prejudice to provisions governing the entry and residence of third-country nationals and their access to employment and to occupation.

(14) In implementing the principle of equal treatment irrespective of racial or ethnic origin, the Community should, in accordance with Article 3(2) of the EC Treaty, aim to eliminate inequalities, and to promote equality between men and women, especially since women are often the victims of multiple discrimination.

(15) The appreciation of the facts from which it may be inferred that there has been direct or indirect discrimination is a matter for national judicial or other competent bodies, in accordance with rules of national law or practice. Such rules may provide in particular for indirect discrimination to be established by any means including on the basis of statistical evidence.

(16) It is important to protect all natural persons against discrimination on grounds of racial or ethnic origin. Member States should also provide, where appropriate and in accordance with their national traditions and practice, protection for legal persons where they suffer discrimination on grounds of the racial or ethnic origin of their members.

(17) The prohibition of discrimination should be without prejudice to the maintenance or adoption of measures intended to prevent or compensate for disadvantages suffered by a group of persons of a particular racial or ethnic origin, and such measures may permit organisations of persons of a particular racial or ethnic origin where their main object is the promotion of the special needs of those persons.

(18) In very limited circumstances, a difference of treatment may be justified where a characteristic related to racial or ethnic origin constitutes a genuine and determining occupational requirement, when the objective is legitimate and the requirement is proportionate. Such circumstances should be included in the information provided by the Member States to the Commission.

(19) Persons who have been subject to discrimination based on racial and ethnic origin should have adequate means of legal protection. To provide a more effective level of protection, associations or legal entities should also be empowered to engage, as the Member States so determine, either on behalf or in support of any victim, in proceedings, without prejudice to national rules of procedure concerning representation and defence before the courts.

(20) The effective implementation of the principle of equality requires adequate judicial protection against victimisation.

(21) The rules on the burden of proof must be adapted when there is a prima facie case of discrimination and, for the principle of equal treatment to be applied effectively, the burden of proof must shift back to the respondent when evidence of such discrimination is brought.

(22) Member States need not apply the rules on the burden of proof to proceedings in which it is for the court or other competent body to investigate the facts of the case. The procedures thus referred to are those in which the plaintiff is not required to prove the facts, which it is for the court or competent body to investigate.

(23) Member States should promote dialogue between the social partners and with non-governmental organisations to address different forms of discrimination and to combat them.

(24) Protection against discrimination based on racial or ethnic origin would itself be strengthened by the existence of a body or bodies in each Member State, with competence to analyse the problems involved, to study possible solutions and to provide concrete assistance for the victims.

(25) This Directive lays down minimum requirements, thus giving the Member States the option of introducing or maintaining more favourable provisions. The implementation of this Directive should not serve to justify any regression in relation to the situation which already prevails in each Member State.

(26) Member States should provide for effective, proportionate and dissuasive sanctions in case of breaches of the obligations under this Directive.

(27) The Member States may entrust management and labour, at their joint request, with the implementation of this Directive as regards provisions falling within the scope of collective agreements, provided that the Member States take all the necessary steps to ensure that they can at all times guarantee the results imposed by this Directive.

(28) In accordance with the principles of subsidiarity and proportionality as set out in Article 5 of the EC Treaty, the objective of this Directive, namely ensuring a common high level of protection against discrimination in all the Member States, cannot be sufficiently achieved by the Member States and can therefore, by reason of the scale and impact of the proposed action, be better achieved by the Community. This Directive does not go beyond what is necessary in order to achieve those objectives,

HAS ADOPTED THIS DIRECTIVE:

CHAPTER I
GENERAL PROVISIONS

Article 1
Purpose

The purpose of this Directive is to lay down a framework for combating discrimination on the grounds of racial or ethnic origin, with a view to putting into effect in the Member States the principle of equal treatment.

Article 2
Concept of discrimination

1. For the purposes of this Directive, the principle of equal treatment shall mean that there shall be no direct or indirect discrimination based on racial or ethnic origin.
2. For the purposes of paragraph 1:

   (a) direct discrimination shall be taken to occur where one person is treated less favourably than another is, has been or would be treated in a comparable situation on grounds of racial or ethnic origin;

   (b) indirect discrimination shall be taken to occur where an apparently neutral provision, criterion or practice would put persons of a racial or ethnic origin at a particular disadvantage compared with other persons, unless that provision, criterion or practice is objectively justified by a legitimate aim and the means of achieving that aim are appropriate and necessary.

3. Harassment shall be deemed to be discrimination within the meaning of paragraph 1, when an unwanted conduct related to racial or ethnic origin takes place with the purpose or effect of violating the dignity of a person and of creating an intimidating, hostile, degrading, humiliating or offensive environment. In this context, the concept of harassment may be defined in accordance with the national laws and practice of the Member States.
4. An instruction to discriminate against persons on grounds of racial or ethnic origin shall be deemed to be discrimination within the meaning of paragraph 1.

Article 3
Scope

1. Within the limits of the powers conferred upon the Community, this Directive shall apply to all persons, as regards both the public and private sectors, including public bodies, in relation to:

   (a) conditions for access to employment, to self-employment and to occupation, including selection criteria and recruitment conditions, whatever the branch of activity and at all levels of the professional hierarchy, including promotion;
   (b) access to all types and to all levels of vocational guidance, vocational training, advanced vocational training and retraining, including practical work experience;
   (c) employment and working conditions, including dismissals and pay;
   (d) membership of and involvement in an organisation of workers or employers, or any organisation whose members carry on a particular profession, including the benefits provided for by such organisations;
   (e) social protection, including social security and healthcare;
   (f) social advantages;
   (g) education;
   (h) access to and supply of goods and services which are available to the public, including housing.

2. This Directive does not cover difference of treatment based on nationality and is without prejudice to provisions and conditions relating to the entry into and residence of third-country nationals and stateless persons on the territory of Member States, and to any treatment which arises from the legal status of the third-country nationals and stateless persons concerned.

Article 4
Genuine and determining occupational requirements

Notwithstanding Article 2(1) and (2), Member States may provide that a difference of treatment which is based on a characteristic related to racial or ethnic origin shall not constitute discrimination where, by reason of the nature of the particular occupational activities concerned or of the context in which they are carried out, such a characteristic constitutes a genuine and determining occupational requirement, provided that the objective is legitimate and the requirement is proportionate.

Article 5
Positive action

With a view to ensuring full equality in practice, the principle of equal treatment shall not prevent any Member State from maintaining or adopting specific measures to prevent or compensate for disadvantages linked to racial or ethnic origin.

Article 6
Minimum requirements

1. Member States may introduce or maintain provisions which are more favourable to the protection of the principle of equal treatment than those laid down in this Directive.
2. The implementation of this Directive shall under no circumstances constitute grounds for a reduction in the level of protection against discrimination already afforded by Member States in the fields covered by this Directive.

CHAPTER II
REMEDIES AND ENFORCEMENT

Article 7
Defence of rights

1. Member States shall ensure that judicial and/or administrative procedures, including where they deem it appropriate conciliation procedures, for the enforcement of obligations under this Directive are available to all persons who consider themselves wronged by failure to apply the principle of equal treatment to them, even after the relationship in which the discrimination is alleged to have occurred has ended.
2. Member States shall ensure that associations, organisations or other legal entities, which have, in accordance with the criteria laid down by their national law, a legitimate interest in ensuring that the provisions of this Directive are complied with, may engage, either on behalf or in support of the complainant, with his or her approval, in any judicial and/or administrative procedure provided for the enforcement of obligations under this Directive.
3. Paragraphs 1 and 2 are without prejudice to national rules relating to time limits for bringing actions as regards the principle of equality of treatment.

Article 8
Burden of proof

1. Member States shall take such measures as are necessary, in accordance with their national judicial systems, to ensure that, when persons who consider

themselves wronged because the principle of equal treatment has not been applied to them establish, before a court or other competent authority, facts from which it may be presumed that there has been direct or indirect discrimination, it shall be for the respondent to prove that there has been no breach of the principle of equal treatment.

2. Paragraph 1 shall not prevent Member States from introducing rules of evidence which are more favourable to plaintiffs.
3. Paragraph 1 shall not apply to criminal procedures.
4. Paragraphs 1, 2 and 3 shall also apply to any proceedings brought in accordance with Article 7(2).
5. Member States need not apply paragraph 1 to proceedings in which it is for the court or competent body to investigate the facts of the case.

Article 9
Victimisation

Member States shall introduce into their national legal systems such measures as are necessary to protect individuals from any adverse treatment or adverse consequence as a reaction to a complaint or to proceedings aimed at enforcing compliance with the principle of equal treatment.

Article 10
Dissemination of information

Member States shall take care that the provisions adopted pursuant to this Directive, together with the relevant provisions already in force, are brought to the attention of the persons concerned by all appropriate means throughout their territory.

Article 11
Social dialogue

1. Member States shall, in accordance with national traditions and practice, take adequate measures to promote the social dialogue between the two sides of industry with a view to fostering equal treatment, including through the monitoring of workplace practices, collective agreements, codes of conduct, research or exchange of experiences and good practices.
2. Where consistent with national traditions and practice, Member States shall encourage the two sides of the industry without prejudice to their autonomy to conclude, at the appropriate level, agreements laying down anti-discrimination rules in the fields referred to in Article 3 which fall within the scope of collective bargaining. These agreements shall respect the minimum requirements laid down by this Directive and the relevant national implementing measures.

Article 12
Dialogue with non-governmental organisations

Member States shall encourage dialogue with appropriate non-governmental organisations which have, in accordance with their national law and practice, a legitimate interest in contributing to the fight against discrimination on grounds of racial and ethnic origin with a view to promoting the principle of equal treatment.

CHAPTER III
BODIES FOR THE PROMOTION OF EQUAL TREATMENT

Article 13

1. Member States shall designate a body or bodies for the promotion of equal treatment of all persons without discrimination on the grounds of racial or ethnic origin. These bodies may form part of agencies charged at national level with the defence of human rights or the safeguard of individuals' rights.
2. Member States shall ensure that the competences of these bodies include:

   – without prejudice to the right of victims and of associations, organisations or other legal entities referred to in Article 7(2), providing independent assistance to victims of discrimination in pursuing their complaints about discrimination,
   – conducting independent surveys concerning discrimination,
   – publishing independent reports and making recommendations on any issue relating to such discrimination.

CHAPTER IV
FINAL PROVISIONS

Article 14
Compliance

Member States shall take the necessary measures to ensure that:
(a) any laws, regulations and administrative provisions contrary to the principle of equal treatment are abolished;
(b) any provisions contrary to the principle of equal treatment which are included in individual or collective contracts or agreements, internal rules of undertakings, rules governing profit-making or non-profit-making associations, and rules governing the independent professions and workers' and employers' organisations, are or may be declared, null and void or are amended.

Article 15
Sanctions

Member States shall lay down the rules on sanctions applicable to infringements of the national provisions adopted pursuant to this Directive and shall take all measures necessary to ensure that they are applied. The sanctions, which may comprise the payment of compensation to the victim, must be effective, proportionate and dissuasive. The Member States shall notify those provisions to the Commission by 19 July 2003 at the latest and shall notify it without delay of any subsequent amendment affecting them.

Article 16
Implementation

Member States shall adopt the laws, regulations and administrative provisions necessary to comply with this Directive by 19 July 2003 or may entrust management and labour, at their joint request, with the implementation of this Directive as regards provisions falling within the scope of collective agreements. In such cases, Member States shall ensure that by 19 July 2003, management and labour introduce the necessary measures by agreement, Member States being required to take any necessary measures to enable them at any time to be in a position to guarantee the results imposed by this Directive. They shall forthwith inform the Commission thereof.
When Member States adopt these measures, they shall contain a reference to this Directive or be accompanied by such a reference on the occasion of their official publication. The methods of making such a reference shall be laid down by the Member States.

Article 17
Report

1. Member States shall communicate to the Commission by 19 July 2005, and every five years thereafter, all the information necessary for the Commission to draw up a report to the European Parliament and the Council on the application of this Directive.
2. The Commission's report shall take into account, as appropriate, the views of the European Monitoring Centre on Racism and Xenophobia, as well as the viewpoints of the social partners and relevant non-governmental organisations. In accordance with the principle of gender mainstreaming, this report shall, inter alia, provide an assessment of the impact of the measures taken on women and men. In the light of the information received, this report shall include, if necessary, proposals to revise and update this Directive.

Article 18
Entry into force

This Directive shall enter into force on the day of its publication in the Official Journal of the European Communities.

Article 19
Addressees

This Directive is addressed to the Member States.

Done at Luxembourg, 29 June 2000.
For the Council
The President
M. Arcanjo
(1) Not yet published in the Official Journal.
(2) Opinion delivered on 18.5.2000 (not yet published in the Official Journal).
(3) Opinion delivered on 12.4.2000 (not yet published in the Official Journal).
(4) Opinion delivered on 31.5.2000 (not yet published in the Official Journal).
(5) OJ L 185, 24.7.1996, p. 5.

Pharmaceuticals Policy and Law 13 (2011) 311–312
DOI 10.3233/PPL-2011-0333
IOS Press

Article 15, Directive 2011/24/EU of the European Parliament and of the Council of 9 March 2011 on the application of patients' rights in cross-border healthcare

Article 15: Cooperation on health technology assessment:

1. The Union shall support and facilitate cooperation and the exchange of scientific information among Member States within a voluntary network connecting national authorities or bodies responsible for health technology assessment designated by the Member States. The Member States shall communicate their names and contact details to the Commission. The members of such a health technology assessment network shall participate in, and contribute to, the network's activities in accordance with the legislation of the Member State where they are established. That network shall be based on the principle of good governance including transparency, objectivity, independence of expertise, fairness of procedure and appropriate stakeholder consultations.
2. The objectives of the health technology assessment network shall be to:
   (a) support cooperation between national authorities or bodies;
   (b) support Member States in the provision of objective, reliable, timely, transparent, comparable and transferable information on the relative efficacy as well as on the short- and long-term effectiveness, when applicable, of health technologies and to enable an effective exchange of this information between the national authorities or bodies;
   (c) support the analysis of the nature and type of information that can be exchanged;
   (d) avoid duplication of assessments.
3. In order to fulfil the objectives set out in paragraph 2, the network on health technology assessment may receive Union aid. Aid may be granted in order to:
   (a) contribute to the financing of administrative and technical support;
   (b) support collaboration between Member States in developing and sharing methodologies for health technology assessment including relative effectiveness assessment;
   (c) contribute to the financing of the provision of transferable scientific information for use in national reporting and case studies commissioned by the network;
   (d) facilitate cooperation between the network and other relevant institutions and bodies of the Union;

(e) facilitate the consultation of stakeholders on the work of the network.

4. The Commission shall, in accordance with the regulatory procedure referred to in Article 16(2), adopt the necessary measures for the establishment, management and transparent functioning of this network.
5. Arrangements for granting the aid, the conditions to which it may be subject and the amount of the aid, shall be adopted in accordance with the regulatory procedure referred to in Article 16(2). Only those authorities and bodies in the network designated as beneficiaries by the participating Member States shall be eligible for Union aid.
6. The appropriations required for measures provided for in this Article shall be decided each year as part of the budgetary procedure.
7. Measures adopted pursuant to this Article shall not interfere with Member States' competences in deciding on the implementation of health technology assessment conclusions and shall not harmonise any laws or regulations of the Member States and shall fully respect the responsibilities of the Member States for the organisation and delivery of health services and medical care.

Pharmaceuticals Policy and Law 13 (2011) 313–314
IOS Press

Author Index Volume 13 (2011)